To Improve Health and Health Care

Volume IX

Stephen L. Isaacs and

James R. Knickman, Editors

Foreword by Risa Lavizzo-Mourey

To Improve Health and Health Care

Volume IX

The Robert Wood Johnson
Foundation Anthology

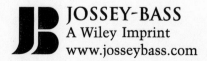

JOSSEY-BASS
A Wiley Imprint
www.josseybass.com

Published by Jossey-Bass
A Wiley Imprint
989 Market Street, San Francisco, CA 94103–1741   www.josseybass.com

Jossey-Bass books and products are available through most bookstores. To contact Jossey-Bass directly call our Customer Care Department within the U.S. at (800) 956–7739, outside the U.S. at (317) 572–3986 or fax (317) 572–4002.

Jossey-Bass also publishes its books in a variety of electronic formats. Some content that appears in print may not be available in electronic books.

ISSN: 1547–3570
ISBN-13: 978–0–7879–8368–0
ISBN-10: 0–7879–8368–3

Printed in the United States of America
FIRST EDITION
PB Printing   10 9 8 7 6 5 4 3 2 1

~ʍ~Table of Contents

–ɯ–Foreword

In keeping our promise to improve the health and health care of all Americans, the Robert Wood Johnson Foundation has developed an impact framework that sets long-, medium-, and short-term objectives for each of our priority areas.[1] Over the past few years, we have become increasingly sophisticated about using all of our resources to achieve these objectives. Although writing checks may be central to our work, we have many other tools at our disposal. Among them are what I call "the five Cs" of effective philanthropy, and the way we employ them can be seen throughout this volume of *The Robert Wood Johnson Foundation Anthology*. The five Cs are:

> ■ *Communicating.* The Foundation has always placed a high value on sharing the results of our work and that of our grantees.[2] Historically, we have emphasized speaking *through* our grantees. Now we are trying to speak *with* our grantees, to be more open in our communications about our own objectives, and to ensure that different audiences get the information they need in a form that they can use and from a source they can trust. The chapter by Susan Krutt and David Morse (Chapter Nine) illustrates the ways in which the Foundation fosters transparency and public accountability. It is complemented by the discussion of Cover the Uninsured Week, a series of communications campaigns designed to keep the uninsured in the public's consciousness, in Robert Rosenblatt's chapter (Chapter Three) on the Foundation's efforts to promote health insurance coverage.

■ *Convening.* The Robert Wood Johnson Foundation has used its prestige and its influence to bring together people who might not ordinarily be in the same room. Perhaps the best recent example is our convening of what we call the "strange bedfellows," discussed in Chapter Three, which brought together health insurance experts with differing positions to see whether they could agree on an approach to covering the uninsured. Although they do not agree on a single approach, the strange bedfellows do agree on some general principles and are continuing to explore options to achieve those principles. On a local scale, under the Free to Grow program, examined by Irene Wielawski in Chapter One, community leaders working with the Head Start program were able to mobilize residents with varied interests who were all concerned about drug and alcohol abuse by young people in their community.

■ *Coordinating.* Although it takes time, requires considerable interpersonal skills, and too often is unrewarded, coordination among multiple stakeholders, especially other funders, is essential. A deft touch is required, and no one has had a defter touch than legendary grantmaker Terrance Keenan, whom we honor in Chapter Eight. In fostering the growth of nurse practitioners and physician assistants, the Foundation, through Keenan, was able to work with and coordinate the efforts of the federal government, academic medical centers, and the nursing profession, among others. As noted by the chapter's author, Digby Diehl, the Foundation, under Keenan's tutelage, developed the Local Initiative Funding Partners program, in which the Robert Wood Johnson Foundation collaborates with local foundations in funding projects that they have identified. Students Run LA, described by Paul Brodeur in Chapter Seven, is a prime example of an effective project funded through the Local Initiative Funding Partners program.

■ *Connecting.* Individual grants become more powerful when one grant builds on another and when the lessons from one project inform others. Continuity and connectivity are often the hallmarks of a well-executed strategy. One of the roles the Foundation plays is connecting the dots—helping grantees see how their own work fits into a larger scheme to meet bigger objectives. In their chapter on healthy aging (Chapter Two), Robin Mockenhaupt, Jane Isaacs Lowe, and Geralyn Graf Magan demonstrate how a group of seemingly disparate grants are in reality elements in a larger strategy, or series of strategies, to improve the health and well-being of older Americans. Similarly, in Chapter Six, Victor Capoccia discusses the evolution of the Foundation's approach to combating drug and alcohol addiction and how individual grants reflect and advance the Foundation's strategies.

■ *Counting.* Monitoring progress by using rigorous and appropriately timed indicators is critical to knowing whether change is taking place. This has long been a hallmark of the Robert Wood Johnson Foundation. Chapters in earlier volumes of the *Anthology* have discussed the Foundation's research and evaluation efforts and the work of grantees such as the Center for Studying Health System Change.[3, 4] In this volume, Marsha Gold and her colleagues Justin White and Erin Fries Taylor at Mathematica Policy Research write about their evaluation of the Medicaid Managed Care Program. The chapter (Chapter Five) illustrates not only the importance of timely assessments but also their value in providing an empirical basis for shifting the emphasis of a program.

The use of the five Cs—combined with a sixth C, cash—can be powerful indeed. Perhaps the best example of the Foundation's using the Cs strategically is its work to reduce smoking between 1990 and the present.[5] The challenge for the Robert Wood Johnson Foundation is to employ all the tools available to it aggressively and purposefully. If we do so, we greatly increase our potential impact and the likelihood of achieving long-lasting returns in health and well-being.

Princeton, New Jersey   Risa Lavizzo-Mourey
October 2005   President and CEO
The Robert Wood Johnson Foundation

Notes

1. See the Foundation's Web site for a listing of the Foundation's portfolios and teams (www.rwjf.org).
2. Karel, F. "'Getting the Word Out': A Foundation Memoir and Personal Journey." *To Improve Health and Health Care 2001: The Robert Wood Johnson Foundation Anthology.* San Francisco: Jossey-Bass, 2001.
3. Knickman, J. "Research as a Foundation Strategy." *To Improve Health and Health Care 2000: The Robert Wood Johnson Foundation Anthology.* San Francisco: Jossey-Bass, 1999.
4. Newbergh, C. "The Health Tracking Initiative." *To Improve Health and Health Care, Vol. VI: The Robert Wood Johnson Foundation Anthology.* San Francisco: Jossey-Bass, 2003.
5. Isaacs, S. L., and Knickman, J. R. "Field Building: Lessons from *The Robert Wood Johnson Foundation Anthology* Series." *Health Affairs,* 2005, *24*(4), 1161–1165.

~⚂~Editors' Introduction: Still Swinging for the Philanthropic Fences?

Since its beginning as a national philanthropy in 1972, the Robert Wood Johnson Foundation has been in the business of fostering social change. To a great extent, whether it has done so or not has been measured by its effect on policy, particularly at the federal level. A Foundation-funded program that leads to a new law or federal funding is considered the equivalent of hitting a home run.

The idea of a philanthropic home run being determined by the federal government's adoption of a new law or policy runs smack into the dominant political and economic belief system of our day—that market forces are the best, and perhaps the only, way to bring about change and that government, especially the federal government, should play a minimal role at best. In this environment, it is fair to ask whether it is reasonable to expect the government to pick up and expand programs that the Foundation started. In baseball parlance, should the Foundation continue to swing for the fences?

The Robert Wood Johnson Foundation Anthology may be able to shed some light on these questions and provide a historical context from which to approach them. The *Anthology* attempts to give readers an understanding of what the Foundation did, why it did it, and what it and others have learned from the experience. Some of what has been learned has to do with the process of going from demonstration projects to policy change and determining when, where, and how it is possible.

In the 1970s, the Robert Wood Johnson Foundation developed a model on which its reputation was based for many years. It funded large demonstration projects—testing an idea or variations of an idea in a number of locations—in the hope that the federal government would adopt the idea, expand it nationwide, and give it continued funding. At a time when people believed that it was government's role to improve their well-being (and that government could do a good job at it), this approach worked in a number of cases.

One of them was the development of an emergency medical services system. Working hand in glove with the federal government at a time when hearses, because of their ample leg room, doubled as ambulances, the Foundation funded demonstration projects that led to the creation of the system of emergency care we have today.[1] It was a home run. Another home run was the establishment of the fields of nurse practitioners and physician assistants. In the early 1970s, with the expectation that national health insurance was just around the corner, the Foundation tested different approaches to making sure that trained personnel would be available to meet the expanded need for care, including a new category of what was called at the time "physician extenders": nurse practitioners and physician assistants. Employing an approach built around demonstration projects but also including a large training component, fellowship programs, and even the formation of professional societies, the Foundation was able to work with and influence the federal government to promote the training and deployment of nurse practitioners and physician assistants.[2]

With the election of Ronald Reagan in 1980, the social and political landscape changed dramatically. Government, especially the federal government, was seen as part of the problem, not part of the solution. The solution was considered, by and large, to be the market. Funding of social programs devolved to the states through block grants, and the likelihood that the federal government would pick up even a successful pilot program diminished significantly.

Still, the Foundation did hit some home runs in the 1980s. One of them was the Health Care for the Homeless Program, funded jointly by the Robert Wood Johnson Foundation and the Pew Charitable Trusts, through which thousands of homeless people received health assessments, services, and referrals through primary care clinicians located in shelters.[3] The program became the template for the hundreds of clinics supported in many cities under the 1987 McKinney Act, the major federal legislative response to homelessness. Another was the AIDS Health Services Program, which between 1986 and 1991 tested a San Francisco community-based model of providing prevention and treatment services. As one of the few foundations funding AIDS services, the Robert Wood Johnson Foundation worked closely with federal officials in planning, implementing, and evaluating the program. The program provided the basis for the Ryan White Act of 1990, the primary federal AIDS legislation.[4]

The change in Washington during the 1980s prompted a rethinking of strategy at the Robert Wood Johnson Foundation. Although Washington remained a focus of the Foundation's efforts, more attention was given to state governments and to organizations outside of government. For example:

- A pilot project in Florida that provided health insurance to children through their schools blossomed into a statewide program that was then picked up by half a dozen other states.[5]

- The Dental Training for the Care of the Handicapped program (which began in the 1970s), in which eleven schools of dentistry incorporated services for handicapped patients in their curricula, led to the American Dental Association's decision to include care for the handicapped as a specific teaching area to be evaluated during accreditation site visits. During the 1980s, programs for instructing dentists in how to treat handicapped patients were started in virtually all of the nation's dental schools.[6]

- In 1978, the Foundation funded an experiment in Elmira, New York, conducted by David Olds, under which trained nurses visited disadvantaged pregnant women during their pregnancy and for a period of time after birth. The experiment was repeated with various permutations in other locations through the 1990s. During this time, the idea of nurse home visitors caught on and was adapted by at least four state governments (Colorado, Hawaii, Missouri, and Oklahoma) and was taken nationwide on a limited basis with funding from Ronald McDonald House charities.[7]

With the fall of the Berlin Wall in 1989 and the collapse of the Soviet Union, the triumph of the market was unchallenged, and social change—in the health field and elsewhere—was built around market forces. In that context, the prospect of health care reform, based on competing managed care organizations, dominated the early 1990s. The possibility of health care reform provided the Foundation with an opportunity to hit a game-winning home run—to parlay the many years of demonstration projects, research, and leadership training it had funded into national health policy. Health care reform at the national level did not, of course, materialize, and its failure was followed by a wave of privatization and consolidation in the industry.

With the potential home run having been caught, as it were, on the outfield warning track, the Foundation turned to a different approach to expand insurance coverage. Rather than trying to catalyze governmental change, it assisted the implementation of existing government policies and programs. The Covering Kids Initiative, for example, supported Medicaid and the State Children's Health Insurance Program by letting families of eligible children know that they could enroll their kids in these government programs.[8] It evolved into Covering Kids & Families, which sought to help states to expand coverage not only to children but to other eligible family members. The Medicaid Managed Care Program attempted, among other things, to improve the way state governments purchased medical services for their Medicaid populations.[9] At the same time, the Foundation did not give up on the idea of promoting affordable health care coverage for all. It funded research on national health insurance options, convened meetings of key players, and to keep the issue alive in the public's consciousness, developed an annual communications campaign called Cover the Uninsured Week.[10]

In the 1990s, the Foundation also developed new strategies to bring about social change in the context of its initiatives to reduce smoking and to improve end-of-life care. Success in these endeavors was measured not only by policy change—although that remained important—but also by changes in the public's attitude and in the behavior of individuals. This called for a wide-ranging approach, one that evolved during the decade.

Tobacco control illustrates the variety of means used by the Foundation. In 1991, at the urging of the Foundation's new president, Steven Schroeder, the board adopted a new goal of reducing the harmful effects and irresponsible use of alcohol, drugs, and tobacco. With respect to smoking, the Foundation gave a series of grants to strengthen the research base and develop a corps of tobacco-policy researchers. Foundation-supported tobacco research focused largely on policy; it funded research, for example, which found that tobacco taxes reduce smoking among teenagers.[11] Complementing its scholarly initiatives, the Foundation funded the Center for Tobacco-Free Kids, a high-profile Washington, D.C., advocacy group, which played a visible role during the tobacco-settlement negotiations and which worked with state organizations to reduce young people's access to cigarettes.[12] It funded the SmokeLess States program, housed in the American Medical Association, which helped state coalitions improve tobacco-control policies, particularly those focused on raising tobacco taxes and reducing secondhand smoke.[13] In its efforts to help people stop smoking, the Foundation funded the development of tobacco-cessation standards, which were adopted by the federal government and used as a tool for businesses to measure the quality of managed care organizations.[14] The breadth of the Foundation's tobacco-control strategy is suggested by its funding of programs targeted at getting pregnant smokers to quit, publicizing the dangers of secondhand smoke, making counseling on tobacco cessation a normal component of preventive care in HMOs, and persuading young people not to start using chewing tobacco. In sum, the Foundation's approach to tobacco-control was a comprehensive one that worked on many levels to bring about policy, systems, and behavioral change.[15]

The Foundation adopted a similar wide-ranging approach toward end-of-life care in the mid-1990s after a large Foundation-funded research study found that the wishes of hospitalized terminally ill patients and their families were routinely ignored.[16] It funded initiatives that developed palliative care programs at major medical centers, increased the attention given to end-of-life care in medical and nursing textbooks, produced a series of articles in medical and nursing journals, and organized coalitions of people working to improve end-of-life care.[17] Its efforts, and those of the Open Society Institute, led the *New York Times* to conclude, "The sharp increase in research on death demonstrates the growing power of philanthropy almost to create an academic field."[18] In fact, the efforts of the two foundations helped advance the field inside and outside of academe.

In the 2000s, it became clear that market forces would continue to dominate political and economic thinking and that the role of government—at least the federal government—would continue to be minimized. The federal government's deficits led budget cutters to apply the axe to social programs, and financially strapped state governments were forced to cut back on social programs such as Medicaid.[19] Not promising terrain for a foundation seeking to be an impetus for government policies or programs directed toward social change!

Under the impetus of Risa Lavizzo-Mourey, who became the president and chief executive officer of the Robert Wood Johnson Foundation in January, 2003, the organization developed an "impact framework" that articulates its long-, medium-, and short-term goals. With one exception—the coverage team that seeks "enactment of a national policy ensuring stable and affordable coverage for all by the year 2010"—the goals set by the Foundation are not targeted toward government. For example, the childhood obesity team, which has set a goal of cutting the percentage of overweight children by half by 2015, plans to do so by working with schools and communities, funding policy research, and developing communications strategies. The disparities team, whose goal is reducing racial and ethnic disparities in the care of targeted diseases by 2008, is working with health care plans, providers, and purchasers.

As Dr. Lavizzo-Mourey notes in her foreword to this volume, the Foundation is now working to bring about social change by using a variety of approaches—what she terms "the five Cs." Not only is it funding research, training, advocacy, public-private partnerships, and communications, it is also using its influence to bring people together, generate partnerships, coordinate a variety of efforts, and give prominence to issues it judges to be important.

A similarly broad strategy has been associated with some of public health's success stories. In areas as different as auto safety, lead-free gasoline, fluoridated water, and tobacco control, change was brought about through a combination of research, advocacy, media attention, and legal and regulatory action.[20]

To answer the question with which we began: Yes, it is possible for the Foundation to hit home runs—to affect major policy change at the federal level. But in the prevailing economic and political circumstances, it is difficult. This does not imply giving up on improving U.S. government policy, but it does signify the need to use all the means available to the Foundation and to consider all levels of government and nongovernment as opportunities to foster social change. Although it is still possible to hit a home run, one can also score with singles, doubles, and deft baserunning.

San Francisco   Stephen L. Isaacs
Princeton, New Jersey   James R. Knickman
October 2005   Editors

Notes

1. Diehl, D. "The Emergency Medical Services Program." In *Anthology 2000* (1999).
2. Keenan, T. "Support of Nurse Practitioners and Physician Assistants." In *Anthology 1998–1999* (1998).
3. Rog, D., and Gutman, M. "The Homeless Families Program: A Summary of Key Findings." In *Anthology 1997* (1997).
4. Bronner, E. "The Foundation and AIDS: Behind the Curve but Leading the Way." In *Anthology, Vol. V* (2002).
5. Holloway, M. "Expanding Health Insurance for Children." In *Anthology 2000* (1999).
6. Brodeur, P. "Improving Dental Care." In *Anthology 2001* (2001).
7. Alper, J. "The Nurse Home Visitation Program." In *Anthology, Vol. V* (2002).
8. Garland, S. "The Covering Kids Communication Campaign." In *Anthology, Vol. VI* (2003).
9. Chapter Five in this volume.
10. Chapter Three in this volume.
11. Gutman, M. A., Altman, D. G., and Rabin, R. L. "Tobacco Policy Research." In *Anthology 1998–1999* (1998).
12. Diehl, D. "The Center for Tobacco-Free Kids and the Tobacco-Settlement Negotiations." In *Anthology, Vol. VI* (2003).

13. Gerlach, K. K., and Larkin M. A. "The SmokeLess States Program." In *Anthology, Vol. VIII* (2005).

14. Orleans, C. T., and Alper, J. "Helping Addicted Smokers Quit: The Foundation's Tobacco-Cessation Programs." In *Anthology, Vol. VI* (2003).

15. Bornemeier, J. "Taking on Tobacco: The Foundation's Assault on Smoking." In *Anthology, Vol. VIII* (2005).

16. Lynn, J. "Unexpected Returns: Insights from SUPPORT." In *Anthology 1997* (1997).

17. Bronner, E. "The Foundation's End-of-Life Programs: Changing the American Way of Death." In *Anthology, Vol. VI* (2003).

18. Miller, J. "When Foundations Chime In: The Issue of Dying Comes to Life." *New York Times,* Nov. 22, 1997.

19. Magnet, M. "The War on the War on Poverty." *Wall Street Journal,* Feb. 25, 2005, p. A18.

20. Isaacs, S. L., and Schroeder, S. A. "Where the Public Good Prevailed." *American Prospect,* June 4, 2001.

–ɯ–Acknowledgments

We wish to express our profound appreciation to the many people whose efforts and commitment to excellence have made this volume of *The Robert Wood Johnson Foundation Anthology* possible.

Within the Robert Wood Johnson Foundation, David Morse has made an invaluable contribution as wise counselor, conscientious editor, and, in this volume, chapter coauthor. Risa Lavizzo-Mourey reviewed every chapter, and we appreciate her insights and suggestions. Katherine Muessig did a remarkable job of gathering materials and assisting authors. She is leaving the Foundation to pursue a masters' degree in public health, and we shall miss her. Molly McKaughan did her usual outstanding job of editing and connecting dots that we otherwise might have missed. Deborah Malloy, Nancy Giordano, Sara Wilkinson, and Sherry DeMarchi provided, once again, near-perfect administrative support. Marilyn Ernst, Carol Owle, Mary Castria, Carolyn Scholer, and Ellen Coyote handled financial matters with competence and goodwill. Hope Woodhead and Barbara Sherwood took care of the book's distribution with great professionalism. Lydia Ryba gave us comfort by checking the accuracy of the dollar amounts and dates of all Foundation grants mentioned in the book. The staff members of the Foundation's information center—Hinda Feige Greenberg, Katherine Flatley, and Mary Beth Kren—were, as usual, outstanding in providing material. A number of people within the Foundation reviewed individual chapters, and we acknowledge the contribution of Nancy Barrand, Linda Bilheimer, David Colby, Katherine Hatton, James Ingram, Carol Kroch, Tracy Orleans, Ann Pomphrey, Judith Stavisky, and Anne Weiss.

C. P. Crow again demonstrated his remarkable skill as an editor, for which we remain grateful. We thank Carolyn Shea for fact checking with such speed and thoroughness, and Lauren MacIntyre for converting hand-marked edited copy into printed text with amazing accuracy. Elizabeth Dawson participated in all aspects of editing and producing the *Anthology,* and we are indebted to her. Greta McKinney performed her bookkeeping duties conscientiously, as usual.

We owe a special debt of gratitude to the *Anthology*'s outside review committee: Susan Dentzer, Frank Karel, William Morrill, Patti Patrizi, and Jonathan Showstack. Their thoughtfulness and sound judgment are vitally important to maintaining the high standard of analysis and writing that characterizes the *Anthology.*

Finally, there are two former leaders of the Robert Wood Johnson Foundation who are frequently interviewed by authors of *Anthology* chapters seeking information about the Foundation's past programs and philosophy. They are quoted frequently in the pages of the *Anthology* series. We would be remiss in not expressing our appreciation to Robert Blendon and Steven Schroeder for their unfailing generosity in sharing their knowledge and expertise with authors and editors alike.

S.L.I. and J.R.K.

To Improve Health and Health Care

Volume IX

From the Foundation's
Vulnerable Populations Portfolio

1

Free to Grow

Irene M. Wielawski

Editors' Introduction

Preventing substance abuse through a preschool program may seem, at first glance, like a strange approach. But this is precisely the strategy behind the Free to Grow program, which has supported fifteen Head Start programs in organizing coalitions of families and social service agencies to reduce substance abuse in their communities. The program's organizers recognized that families with young children wanted their children to grow up in a safe, nurturing environment and that Head Start was a natural locus for parents and social service agencies to collaborate on projects that would improve the life of the community and ultimately reduce substance abuse.

One reason for using local Head Start programs to house Free to Grow was the hope that if the coalitions proved successful, the national Head Start program might adopt the program and continue its funding. This hope has not been realized, however, as financial belt-tightening has hit the Head Start program nationally. Ironically, the criminal justice agencies—rather than health, education, or substance abuse agencies—have shown the most interest in the model.

Free to Grow is one of a number of initiatives that the Robert Wood Johnson Foundation has funded to address drug and alcohol addiction—initiatives that are discussed elsewhere in this volume.[1] In some ways, Free to Grow is similar in approach to Fighting Back, another large Foundation-supported effort built around the development of community anti-drug coalitions.[2] However, Free to Grow's more general community development approach and its home in the Head Start program distinguish it from Fighting Back. The author of this chapter, Irene Wielawski, a former investigative reporter for the *Los Angeles Times* and now a freelance journalist specializing in health and health care issues, is a frequent contributor to the *Anthology* series.

1. Capoccia, V. "The Evolution of the Robert Wood Johnson Foundation's Approach to Alcohol and Drug Addiction." *To Improve Health and Health Care, Vol. IX: The Robert Wood Johnson Foundation Anthology.* San Francisco: Jossey-Bass, 2006.

2. Wielawski, I. "The Fighting Back Program." *To Improve Health and Health Care, Vol. VII: The Robert Wood Johnson Foundation Anthology.* San Francisco: Jossey-Bass, 2004.

—ᴡ— N o one in Owensboro, Kentucky, expected Foust Elementary School to set records for achievement. With a student body of mostly poor children from the city's crime-ridden West End, Foust had consistently ranked near the bottom on statewide reading, writing, and science proficiency examinations for fourth-graders.

In 1999, the Foust students showed some improvement in their scores, but not enough to alter local opinion. In 2000, the scores went up again, but some people still saw the improvement as a statistical fluke. An even bigger jump came in 2001, and the next year, and the year after that. By 2004, no one could dispute the validity of Foust's upward trend. In writing improvement alone, Foust had reached the top 5 percent of schools statewide—and was poised to meet the proficiency goals of the Kentucky Department of Education six years ahead of schedule. Heralding the achievement, the Owensboro *Messenger-Inquirer* called Foust's 2004 gains "huge."[1] A Kentucky Department of Education spokeswoman said they were nothing short of "amazing."

Why amazing? Because the Foust student body contains every socioeconomic handicap that historically correlates with subpar school performance—as well as with substance abuse and other harmful behavior later in life. Extreme poverty is one of these handicaps. In 2004, some 96 percent of the Foust students qualified for federal free or reduced-price school lunches, compared with an average in Kentucky schools of 52 percent. Many of the students also come from single-parent homes in neighborhoods riven by street violence, drug dealing, and other social ills. They may have little supervision during nonschool hours, and are more likely than privileged children to come to school anxious and exhausted. Given such conditions, "amazing" is hardly too strong a description of the Foust students' achievement.

Accounting for it, however, is more complicated, given the myriad influences on children's ability and their readiness to learn. Studies show that the conditions of early childhood have far-reaching consequences not only for achievement in school but also for later in life. So-called environmental risk factors can predispose a child to harmful behavior such as drug and alcohol abuse. The risks identified by social scientists include severe poverty, transience, substance and other abuse in the home, neighborhood mayhem, and early school failure. Mitigating these risks are so-called protective factors that augment children's resilience in the face of adversity. Protective factors include high intelligence and positive emotional bonds within the family and the neighborhood and among peers.[2]

Children born into difficult circumstances aren't without resources. Many public and private agencies share a mission to help them. The work of these agencies, however, is often piecemeal, because of numerous poorly coordinated and sometimes competitive institutional mandates and funding streams. Professionals within these agencies—teachers, social workers, pediatricians, police officers, and youth counselors, to name a few—commonly express frustration at being able to do only part of the job. The question naturally arises: might coordinating these risk-reduction activities across the agencies involved while simultaneously working to build resilience yield greater long-term success?

This was the challenge—and the ambition—of a wide-ranging anti-drug-and-alcohol experiment launched by the Robert Wood Johnson Foundation in partnership with the federal Head Start preschool program. Called Free to Grow: Head Start Partnerships to Promote Substance-Free Communities, it was authorized in 1992 for testing in six pilot communities and expanded in 2000 to fifteen demonstration sites. The Foundation committed more than $14 million over thirteen years: $5.4 million for the five-year pilot phase, $1 million for a process evaluation of phase one, $4 million for the four-year demonstration phase (through 2005), and another $4 million for evaluation of the demonstration phase. Additional support for the program comes from the Doris Duke Charitable Foundation ($2.9 million) and for the evaluation from the Office of Juvenile Justice and Delinquency Prevention of the U.S. Department of Justice ($1 million).

Free to Grow provides no direct service to Head Start youngsters. Instead, it brings together broad-based community partners in efforts to strengthen families and communities, thereby addressing the young child's overall environment. The program is based on a body of research that identifies family and neighborhood characteristics that can heighten or moderate the risk of substance abuse and other harms. Guided by this research, Free to Grow fosters partnerships among existing community and family service organizations, police, and government agencies to mitigate the threats to children and uses the structural framework of Head Start to reach needy families and neighborhoods.

The program defines threat broadly. Obvious threats—addicted or abusive family members, for example, or roving street gangs—share attention with subtler threats, such as vermin-infested housing, lack of supervised after-school programs, and hostility between neighborhood residents and police. Free to Grow, as a result, stands apart from traditional substance abuse prevention efforts such as DARE, through which police officers visit schools to teach children about the dangers of drugs, alcohol, and tobacco. Many of Free to Grow's activities are only tangentially related to substance abuse; the program's portfolio includes initiatives against crime, negligent landlords, unemployment, adult illiteracy, language barriers, even traffic problems. Residents in one target community credit Free to Grow with helping them get stop signs installed at a dangerous intersection. That the signs had no immediate impact on the local methamphetamine trade is beside the point. The theory of Free to Grow holds that when impoverished families and communities believe they can change things for the better—like making an intersection safer, for instance—the neighborhood will gather the resolve to purge itself of other problems.

Judith Jones, clinical professor at the Mailman School of Public Health at Columbia University and founding director of the National Center for Children in Poverty, is director of the Free to Grow national program office. The principal investigator of a national evaluation of the program's fifteen-site demonstration phase is Mark Wolfson of the Department of Public Health Sciences at Wake Forest University School of Medicine. The evaluation is funded through 2006. This isn't long enough to answer the question of whether Free to Grow interventions adopted during the preschool years increased protective factors sufficiently to alter patterns of substance abuse during the teen years. Instead, the evaluation is tracking change in the mixture of family and community risk and protective factors across Free to Grow sites, and comparing these sites with comparable communities whose Head Start agencies did not participate in Free to Grow.

—ɯ— The Genesis of Free to Grow

How an undertaking as diffuse as Free to Grow came to be embraced in 1992 by the Robert Wood Johnson Foundation and the signature government antipoverty program, Head Start, is best understood in historical context. America's drug problem was major news at the time—a problem that had been made worse by crack cocaine's devastating impact on inner-city families and neighborhoods during the 1980s. At Head Start, teachers were seeing that impact in the behavior of three- and four-year-olds in their classrooms—and on Head Start's prospects for readying these children for kindergarten. At the Robert Wood Johnson Foundation, meanwhile, staff members were scrambling to respond to a new president's call for innovative approaches to reduce the harm from alcohol, tobacco, and drug abuse.

Steven Schroeder, who served as Foundation president from July 1990 until December 2002, remembers being asked, during interviews for the job in 1989, what he would do differently. "I said, 'Well your mission is health and health care, but you are only doing health care.'" Schroeder suggested adding substance abuse initiatives to the mission for two reasons. First, drugs, alcohol, and tobacco are harmful to health, which puts substance-abuse interventions squarely within the mission to improve health and health care. Second, the field needed innovation. Private philanthropies, Schroeder argued, have greater latitude than government "to try some new approaches."

As president, Schroeder was given the go-ahead. He launched a re-structuring of funding priorities to prune the Foundation's many health improvement ventures to only those defined by three broad categories: access to health care, chronic illness, and the new one: substance abuse. An immediate problem was lack of in-house expertise in alcohol and drug abuse prevention and treatment. Staff members schooled in other disciplines headed to the library to get up to speed. Free to Grow was one of several prevention-oriented initiatives to come out of this era. Its chief architect was Marjorie Gutman, a social psychologist and, at the time, a Foundation program officer. She worked with Nancy Kaufman, who had recently joined the Foundation as a vice president, on early conceptual versions of Free to Grow.

"We wanted to do something for high-risk kids, and we wanted to get in earlier than the usual time, adolescence," Gutman recalls. "The theory was that if you could alter the trajectory early enough, it might make a difference." But how to reach these high-risk youngsters, and at what age? Gutman was inspired by research from the mental health field on pediatric emotional and behavioral disorders (a risk factor for substance abuse), some of which emerged as early as preschool.

"Suddenly we thought, 'Oh my gosh, Head Start!'" Gutman recalls. "The Foundation is big on infrastructure, and our challenge was to get this idea past the exploration stage. Head Start seemed like it would maximize a lot of potential. There was a huge national infrastructure, and Head Start's mission—in addition to a focus on early childhood education—encompasses health and family and neighborhood."

From Head Start's point of view, Free to Grow was "a natural partner," says Sarah Greene, president and chief executive officer of the Head Start Association, a not-for-profit organization that supports and serves as an advocate for the 1,670 local Head Start agencies serving 900,000 low-income preschoolers nationwide. The concept fit with Head Start's holistic approach to children and families as well as with an operating style that sought partnerships with existing social and health service agencies to meet preschoolers' needs. Free to Grow's designers hoped to build the network of partnerships so family and community needs might also be met. A rough outline emerged from discussions between Head Start and Robert Wood Johnson Foundation staff. "One of our local responsibilities is to assess the family and make whatever changes are necessary to assist the child and that family," Greene says. "The Robert Wood Johnson Foundation's goal to rid these neighborhoods of drug abuse was a perfect fit for what we do, because so many of our children grow up in neighborhoods stricken with violence."

A 1992 article published in *Psychological Bulletin* provided the theoretical framework for Free to Grow.[3] It described how prevention science could be applied to reduce substance abuse by teenagers and young adults. Essentially, it outlined an approach similar to the comprehensive public health measures typically deployed against infectious disease. Direct action to contain or neutralize the threatening bio-organism is accompanied by efforts to boost public protection, such as vaccination, better diet, improved hygiene, and so on. In the context of reducing illegal drug abuse, this comprehensive approach means targeting not only drug dealers but also conditions in neighborhoods—abandoned buildings, for example— that attract the drug trade, and conditions in peer groups and families that may predispose individuals to substance abuse. Richard Catalano, Jr., of the University of Washington, coauthor of the 1992 study, who has published widely in the field of substance abuse prevention, is chairman of Free to Grow's evaluation advisory panel.

—◊— Building the Structure

Because the main ideas behind Free to Grow were untested, the program's leaders decided to roll them out in distinct phases, refining assumptions along the way. "There really was no research to support this," says Judith Jones, the national program director, who brought many years of work with disadvantaged communities and children to her leadership. "We knew we were going to have to wait until the Head Start kids were teenagers to see if any of this works."

The first phase got under way in 1994 with two-year grants of about $300,000 each to six Head Start programs in urban and rural settings chosen to develop models to test Free to Grow's prevention theory. By 1996, five of the sites showed sufficient promise to be awarded three-year implementation grants of approximately $600,000 each. The sites were Rio Piedras, Puerto Rico; Compton, California; Colorado Springs, Colorado; Washington Heights, New York; and Owensboro, Kentucky, where Foust Elementary School is located.

The sites came up with various strategies to strengthen families and communities. Strategies to strengthen families included assessment and case management, referral as needed to counseling or treatment, parent education classes, peer mentoring and support groups, and transition assistance for families moving from Head Start, which is very hands-on, to elementary schools, which are less so. Strategies to strengthen communities included organizing residents and existing groups to survey neighborhood needs (as opposed to bringing in outsiders to do the job), working together on solutions, building leadership skills, and fostering partnerships among existing local agencies. The partnerships were crucial, since Free to Grow by itself has no services to offer. From the outset, program leaders wanted to avoid the pitfall of many grant-funded programs that serve poor people for a while and then disappear when the money runs out. As a consequence, collaborations in this pilot phase varied tremendously from site to site, depending on available local resources and the quality of existing relationships. Across sites, however, two partners jumped out from the pilot phase as critically important assets: schools and police. The schools weren't surprising, since they share Head Start's education mission. But the interest and the enthusiasm of police was unexpected. As the program played out, police would surpass local educators as Free to Grow's strongest allies and advocates. The finding in the pilot phase was strong enough for the Foundation and national Free to Grow leaders to require police and school representatives as "core partners" in planning, governance, budget allocation, and implementation of demonstration projects.

The Foundation solicited applications for phase 2—the "demonstration phase"—in early 2000, with grant awards made to the selected Head Start programs in June 2001. Conceptually, Free to Grow now had more rigid guidelines. Besides requiring schools and police on the governance team, the call for proposals "strongly recommended" that applicant Head Start agencies recruit their local substance abuse treatment agency. In addition, these partners were suggested:

- Family guidance agencies
- Mental health agencies
- Community-based prevention coalitions and community action groups
- Employment training programs
- Local youth service organizations

Winning applicants were to receive roughly $200,000 from the Foundation over four years, and the grant money had to be matched by $50,000 annually from local sponsors or extra Head Start dollars. The first year of the demonstration phase was to be spent in training, developing action plans, and networking with residents and partners. The next three years (2002–2005) were to be devoted to implementation. To channel the potential range of activities to be carried out by grantees, the call for proposals summarized effective interventions from the first-phase pilot sites, and required demonstration sites to select from these models and adapt strategies to their localities.

One hundred twenty-five Head Start agencies sent letters of intent to apply, and forty-seven of them followed up with full applications. Of these, the Foundation selected eighteen applicants to receive one-year development grants to be used for capacity building, community assessment, and program start-up. In June 2002, the Foundation selected fifteen sites for funding of the implementation stage: Phoenix, Arizona; Orange, California; New Britain, Connecticut; Delray Beach, Florida; Wailuku, Hawaii; Jenkins, Kentucky; Franklin, Louisiana; Lexington Park, Maryland; Lincoln, Nebraska; Laguna, New Mexico; Tulsa, Oklahoma; Hermiston, Oregon; Dallas, Texas; Barre, Vermont; and Wausau, Wisconsin.

—୴୴— Themes and Variations

Even though phase-two sites were required to adapt model interventions from phase one, the sites still had considerable latitude. It could hardly be otherwise with an undertaking aimed at encouraging and providing tools for poor families and communities to "take ownership" of their destinies, in the oft-used phrase of Free to Grow leaders. Moreover, the conditions Free to Grow has sought to alleviate differ from one community to another. Evidence of this abounded at the program's 2004 annual meeting, at which grantees showed videos of project undertakings ranging from housing code enforcement campaigns to community picnics to a unique campaign in Wisconsin to overturn a state law that permits children accompanied by parents to drink in taverns. The limitless possibilities of environmental improvement in deprived families and communities seem to infect the participants, leading to field operations that expand in ever-widening concentric circles around the target problem. How that plays out is best seen in the experiences of individual sites. Three examples are offered, one from the 1994–1999 pilot phase and two from the current 2001–2005 demonstration phase.

Owensboro, Kentucky

Owensboro's Head Start program, a department of Audubon Area Community Services, was one of the original grantees in Free to Grow's pilot phase. Although Free to Grow officially wrapped up here in 1999, Owensboro has since found the means to incorporate some elements into the local Head Start infrastructure while sustaining several of the partnerships developed under Free to Grow.

Audubon Area Head Start has a bigger operation than most Free to Grow grantees, with a total of 1,702 preschool slots in fifty-six centers. Its headquarters are in Owensboro, which is western Kentucky's largest city (population 54,000), but jurisdiction extends well beyond the city limits into many of the towns of surrounding agricultural counties as far south as the Tennessee border. Tobacco is the local crop and a major source of employment on farms and in processing facilities like the huge, windowless U.S. Smokeless Tobacco Company plant in Hopkinsville, a two-hour drive from Owensboro, in rural Christian County.

The mayor of Hopkinsville, Rich Liebe, speaks proudly of landing big companies like U.S. Smokeless Tobacco, saying the move from a purely farming base to an industrial and agribusiness economy has enabled Hopkinsville to respond better to the residents' needs, particularly those of poor families who depend on public services. Colorful evidence of this is found in the playgrounds of local housing projects and community parks: new, crayon-bright swings and slides and climbing equipment dominate what once were litter-strewn congregating spots for lowlifes, according to officials and local residents. As a result, tobacco doesn't receive the disapproval here that it might at the Robert Wood Johnson Foundation or Free to Grow's national headquarters in New York City or a Free to Grow site where tobacco has no impact on livelihood and the tax base. But if tobacco quietly drops out of the group of anti–substance abuse initiatives here, it in no way diminishes local officials' enthusiastic embrace of partnership with the Owensboro Free to Grow project, which chose Hopkinsville to test community-strengthening strategies.

It was in Hopkinsville that getting the four-way stop began changing attitudes in a part of town where local government and police were rarely seen as the residents' allies. East First Street and Greenville Road had for years been a murderous intersection bordering the Rozell housing project, a tidy, two-story, clapboard complex for low-income families, most of them African American. Diagonally across Greenville Road is a small convenience store where children from the project buy snacks after school, and where elderly residents without cars get their groceries. Because Greenville Road is a major thoroughfare in Hopkinsville, crossing on foot was always a breathless experience. Trying to get across or to turn into Greenville from East First was equally tough in a car.

"My best friend was in a car wreck there," says Arma Jean Rawlins, a Head Start classroom aide who lives in the Rozell project. Through Free to Grow, Rawlins got involved with a neighborhood group that was formed to work with police and city officials on several festering neighborhood issues, among them the intersection and the dilapidated playgrounds. "I didn't know what to expect, but we learned to stick together and keep pushing," says Rawlins, whose Free to Grow community work led to her appointment to the Hopkinsville Housing Authority.

Rawlins credits Mary Lester, Free to Grow's community outreach worker, with keeping her residents' committee focused when setbacks and bureaucracy sapped their energy and their confidence that "powerful people" would respond. Lester herself is a Free to Grow success story. A single mother of four and a Head Start parent, she never envisioned herself in the job she's still doing, six years after Free to Grow officially expired here. "Oh, no, I did not speak in front of people, no way," she says, recalling her reaction to being chosen for the outreach worker job.

Mayor Liebe calls Lester "a circuit-rider preacher" for community action. "I began to think she was working for me, she was popping into my office so often with this idea or that," he says. "There's a genuineness in Mary to help which I responded to." Lester acted as the communication link between Rawlins's neighborhood group and the mayor's office. She also helped residents figure out who, for example, they needed to petition at the Kentucky Highway Department for the traffic light they wanted at First and Greenville. She showed them how to research such questions, using the Internet to locate the relevant branch of state government, addresses, phone numbers, and procedures for filing requests. It seemed that victory was imminent when state engineers showed up one day to survey the intersection. But celebration turned out to be premature. In their report, the engineers said traffic volume wasn't sufficient to meet the state threshold for stoplights. Mayor Liebe was as irate as residents of the Rozell complex. More letters and petitions, backed by the mayor's office and the police department, went out in the mail—this time addressed to county officials. It was the residents who came up with this strategic end run, having discovered in their research that while red-yellow-green traffic lights were controlled by the state, county government ruled stop signs and blinking lights. Today, four stop signs and a blinking light have improved perceptions of safety in the neighborhood, and stand as evidence to residents that they're not as powerless as they once believed.

Similar organizing efforts in Owensboro led to improvements in the city's West End, where crack cocaine brought mayhem in the early 1990s. A surge in violent crime, with four drug-related murders in a city accustomed to no more than a single murder a year, brought many calls for action. Under the banner of Free to Grow, West End residents welcomed a community policing program to rid the neighborhood of drug dealers and their customers. The shared objective provided an opportunity to ease long-standing tension between West End residents and local police, according to Lieutenant Ken Bennett, who headed the community police unit. "It was an eye-opener," he says. "As law enforcement officers, we have zero tolerance for drugs, of course, but we found out there were other issues the community was concerned about that are quality-of-life issues, like cracking down on boom boxes and cars roaring through at two in the morning, getting action on abandoned buildings to board them up, getting the trash picked up."

Two lessons emerged from the improved dialogue between police and residents. Police officers discovered that most West End residents were law-abiding. The residents learned that they had to be part of the solution; police couldn't do it all. This led to vital communication. Residents monitored license plates and confided to police officers where they believed illegal activity was taking place. Police followed up, showing residents that they were genuinely concerned about their welfare. It is interesting that it was traffic control tools and enforcement that brought noticeable improvement. These included speed bumps and yellow no-parking paint on curbs within housing projects so drug dealers could be ticketed for doing business out of their cars, and customers driving in from elsewhere could be rousted. "We knew we weren't going to completely stop the drug trade, but we were not going to allow an open-air marketplace in Owensboro," Bennett says.

The fact that Free to Grow offers no services and presents itself solely as a liaison between Head Start's families and the larger community helps cement partnerships with agencies that otherwise might not have collaborated because of turf or other competitive concerns, says Aubrey Nehring, director of Audubon Area Head Start and a member of Free to Grow's national advisory committee. In implementing the Free to Grow pilot project, Nehring needed to hire new staff members, such as Mary Lester for community outreach, because traditional Head Start doesn't extend that far. But the other part of Free to Grow, family advocacy, has been part of Head Start's structure since the program began in 1965. So all Nehring had to do was train existing staff members in the theory of risk and protective factors, and in Free to Grow strategies for strengthening families. This led to a significant revision of Head Start's family assessment questionnaire; the model questionnaire developed in Owensboro is one of the phase-one strategies that has largely been adopted by phase-two sites. Head Start caseworkers now ask pointed questions about alcohol and drug use in the home, violence, child abuse, and mental illness, and also look at family strengths that can be built upon. "The mentality of Head Start here before Free to Grow was that every child and every family was equal and got the same level of service," Nehring says. "We'd always done family needs assessments, but we never had an objective scale to quantify different levels of need and then tailor services to that need." Where some Head Start parents need relatively simple referrals for job training, perhaps, or English classes, others might be overwhelmed by problems so severe—homelessness, substance abuse, depression or other illness—that they need urgent attention from multiple agencies and frequent caseworker visits.

As a preschool program, Head Start's relationship with needy families lasts at best two years. This is a short period to turn around addiction or mental illness, so changes to the family assessment questionnaire led logically to more dynamic partnerships with local agencies that could help. In Owensboro and elsewhere, Head Start employees and personnel at partner agencies repeatedly talk of discovering job overlap and mutually useful services that they never knew existed. These collaborative relationships exist both at the individual level—between a special education teacher at the local elementary school and a Head Start family advocate, say—and among agencies. In Owensboro, one lasting result is a dynamic collaboration between Head Start, local schools, and River Valley Behavioral Health, a federally funded mental health and substance abuse treatment agency serving seven western Kentucky counties. "Pre-Free to Grow, those relationships were tangential," says Gary Hall, River Valley's executive director. "Post-Free to Grow, they've become more formalized. We're more invested in each other's programs because we see a common mission."

New Britain, Connecticut

Forty years ago, New Britain was widely regarded as the jewel of Connecticut's Precision Valley—so-called for the many factories and skilled metalworkers who turned out machine and hand tools, springs, bearings, and other products for the world market. It was a destination for immigrants and post–World War II refugees seeking the American Dream. Many of them realized it, building single- and multifamily homes in New Britain and using generous blue-collar wages to send their children to college.

The factories of that era are mostly shuttered today, victims of new technology and outsourcing to countries with cheaper labor. Better-paid skilled work has been replaced by minimum-wage service jobs. The boom years of the 1990s largely bypassed New Britain, and residents and community leaders see few prospects on the horizon. They're surrounded instead by the evidence of economic decline: derelict buildings, bare-bones city services, and overcrowded schools. Fewer than half of New Britain children attend preschool, compared with Connecticut's average of 75 percent, and school achievement significantly lags behind state and national norms, according to Merrill Gay, executive director of the New Britain Discovery Collaborative. Within this context, the local Head Start program has been fighting to add preschool spots.

New Britain continues to attract immigrants, however. Hispanics have moved into neighborhoods once inhabited by Polish and other Eastern European refugees. With the new demographics come some worrisome trends. "Half the kids under age five are growing up in one-parent homes, and 62 percent qualify for free or reduced lunch at school," Gay says. Families in New Britain's poor neighborhoods are also moving more than they used to, causing stress on children and making it difficult for schools, social agencies, and even programs like Free to Grow to establish protective beachheads. "If children are moving every six months because the family is getting evicted, they lose even the stability of being in a consistent school setting," Gay says. On top of this dislocation is the isolation that comes from not being able to speak English, further separating these families from the larger community and its resources. Compared with Owensboro, Kentucky, which has a stronger economy and a relatively homogeneous population, New Britain's Free to Grow program has had to build its framework almost from scratch. In 2004, for example, two years into the implementation period, Head Start and local school officials were still working on a system to share information on Head Start children so that the results of developmental assessments routinely performed at Head Start, such as vision, hearing, and cognitive tests, could inform the next set of teachers. Owensboro already had this in place when the Free to Grow pilot was launched there in 1994.

Nevertheless, Head Start staff and residents in New Britain credit Free to Grow networking strategies with quality-of-life improvements that they say could not have been accomplished through Head Start alone. For one, the North Oak neighborhood targeted by Free to Grow now has a police substation as well as a community center, which opened in 2003 in what was an abandoned Ukrainian social club. After extensive renovations, two new Head Start classrooms recently opened in the community center. This is a boon in a neighborhood where mothers were taking buses to get children to more distant Head Start facilities. The community center is seen as a safe venue for neighborhood gatherings and a convenient location for recreational and educational programs for adults and children. Two new Girl Scout troops hold meetings there.

Three blocks up from the community center is the police substation, a one-story clapboard cottage that is easily the prettiest property in the neighborhood, with fresh paint, a well-trimmed lawn, and attractive landscaping. This handsome substation is a source of pride to local residents and a symbol of the city's commitment to their well-being. Officers assigned to the North Oak substation hope to become a familiar presence, both as reassurance to residents and business owners and as a warning to potential lawbreakers. A prominent Free to Grow partner is New Britain Weed and Seed, part of a national program established in 1991 by the U.S. Department of Justice as a multi-agency approach to crime prevention and neighborhood improvement. Its long-range goals are remarkably similar to those of Free to Grow, although framed in the language of law enforcement rather than that of family and community empowerment. A government brochure describing the program reads:

> The goals of Weed and Seed are to control violent crime, drug trafficking, and drug-related crime in targeted high-crime neighborhoods and provide a safe environment free of crime and drug use for residents. The Weed and Seed strategy brings together federal, state, and local crime-fighting agencies, social service providers, representatives of the public and private sectors, prosecutors, business owners, and neighborhood residents under the shared goal of weeding out violent crime and gang activity while seeding in social services and economic revitalization.[4]

With Weed and Seed focused on the same New Britain neighborhood as Free to Grow, partnership is a given, says Weed and Seed coordinator MaryAnn Drury. "If you look at three-, four-, and five-year-olds in poor inner-city families, they often aren't eating," she says. "Teenagers are having babies. The parents often have no education themselves so they can't really help their child with homework." Weed and Seed workers turn to the partnership when they come across problems police don't have the time or the expertise to handle, such as vermin-infested housing. "You go into some of these homes, they've got bread stapled to the walls so the cockroaches won't bite the kids," says Officer Steven King, who works out of the North Oak substation and is also the New Britain Police Department's representative to Free to Grow and Weed and Seed, as well as a DARE officer in city schools.

Partly because King wears so many hats and partly because community improvement work doesn't fit neatly into a nine-to-five schedule, his workday routinely stretches into the evening—a common experience for Free to Grow activists and their partners. King attends neighborhood gatherings to keep up with what's happening as well as to put himself where residents shy of police might open up. One evening last fall, he stood for two hours in the community center hallway, relegated there because of an overflow crowd in the center's main meeting room. The occasion was a visit by Representative Nancy L. Johnson, a Republican congresswoman from Connecticut's fifth district, who was on a swing through her hometown and wanted to see the community center and meet her newest constituents. She's also a fan of Free to Grow, seeing it as an interesting experiment in bringing coordination and efficiency to disparate social services. "I am interested in a far more integrated system to deliver services to families that are struggling," she says. "To deliver services effectively, you have to think about health care, education, job training, substance-abuse treatment, everything all at once."

Despite Johnson's enthusiasm for Free to Grow, the project director, Elizabeth Donnellan, had fretted about turnout for the congresswoman's visit. Many North Oak residents work several jobs. Others are afraid to venture out after dark. For weeks beforehand, Donnellan had talked up the meeting with Head Start parents and assigned Elena Trueworthy, the project's bilingual community worker, to spread the word to Spanish-speaking families. Twenty minutes before the scheduled start time, Donnellan paced up and down the hallway, worried that no one would come. In the meeting room, volunteers laid out platters of rice and beans and shredded pork for those who might arrive directly from work. People began to trickle in, some holding babies and trailed by school-age children too young to leave at home. The trickle became a stream. By the time Johnson arrived, the center was so crowded she could barely get through the doorway of the meeting room. One by one, people stood up to tell Johnson why Head Start and Free to Grow were important to them. The father of two young elementary school boys made his presentation in halting English, aided by people sitting near him who suggested words when he faltered. "I proud because my son, he earn, how say it, certificate, Student of Month, in school, and he was Head Start kid." Donnellan slid out of the room, taking refuge in the hall so she could cry unnoticed. "This is Free to Grow," she sobbed happily to Officer King. "I've been with Head Start for twenty-five years and I never could have imagined this, all these people coming here, coming together."

Wailuku, Hawaii

The government seat of Maui, Hawaii, is situated at the northern end of the island in the town of Wailuku. County offices are here, as are headquarters for many agencies, including Maui Economic Opportunity, the parent organization of the island's Head Start program. Also in Wailuku is Kahekili Terrace, a fifty-six-unit public housing project for low-income, mostly native Hawaiian families. Children growing up here experience the underside of the world-renowned paradise that draws millions of tourists to luxurious beachfront resorts, golf courses, and all manner of waterfront recreation. There are no ocean vistas at Kahekili Terrace—just an irrigation ditch running along the project's access road. Before Free to Grow, that road was choked with cars, some of them abandoned, some serving as temporary shelter for vagrants, while others served as the business offices of dealers in crystal methamphetamine, known locally as ice. Ice has swept through Hawaii in recent years, with devastating consequences. Officials at the Maui Community Correctional Center estimate that 90 percent of the inmates have drug habits, and many are incarcerated for drug-related crimes.

Ernie Ramos, a Kahekili resident, says he lost his brother to ice. Having watched his brother's decline, Ramos was upset to see drug dealers operating under the windows of project residents. Still, he questioned what he personally could do about it. The dealers were known to have weapons; Ramos's brother had been shot to death. Ramos kept these feelings to himself until one night at a meeting of project residents, when they surged into the open and into a call for action. The trigger was a suggestion by the housing project manager that residents didn't care about the deteriorating conditions at Kahekili. "I told him it was insulting to say that we didn't care," Ramos recalls. His friend Sharon Fernandez was upset, too, but more about the fact that residents were so cowed. "If we are going to be afraid, it is only going to get worse," she told the group. This was the beginning of the residents' patrol at Kahekili Terrace, an effort spearheaded by the Maui Police Department and the local housing authority and supported by Free to Grow. Fernandez and Ramos were the patrol's first members. "We're not vigilantes," Fernandez explains. "We just observe and let the police know what's going on. It's peer pressure sometimes, like saying to people sitting outside and drinking and being loud, 'These are your neighbors, why're you acting like that?'"

Residents say the patrol has led to significant improvement at Kahekili. Thanks to an aggressive ticketing and towing campaign by Maui Police Sergeant Jamie Becraft and Officer Craig Bajadali, the community policing team assigned to Kahekili, cars no longer park along the access road, and graffiti and litter are gone as well. Residents say the project feels safer now, and the improvements have given them an impetus for new projects. One is a computer lab—the computers have already been donated—so that children from the project don't lag behind more affluent classmates in computer skills required for success in school. Another is an after-school homework program, sponsored by the Boys and Girls Club, called "power hour," which Kahekili Terrace will have on-site. Children participating in the program earn points toward rewards; the Maui version is an airplane trip to Big Island for diving and spear fishing. Kahekili Terrace also has its own Head Start classroom, opened as part of Free to Grow's community-strengthening investment.

Getting the OK to open that classroom, however, illustrates the difficulties that can arise in adopting what seems like a straightforward Free to Grow strategy. The problem at Kahekili Terrace was fire truck access.

The classroom was too far from existing hydrants to get a school occupancy permit. Clearing the regulatory tangle took two years, according to the Head Start director, Lyn McNeff. In the end, Head Start paid for the installation of a hydrant close enough to the classroom to satisfy safety requirements.

Maui's Free to Grow project also sponsors programs to enable children and incarcerated mothers to spend a day together outside the prison setting—an undertaking that requires partnership with the Maui Community Correctional Center. The project is also working to address the lack of affordable housing for island residents. These are all efforts to address environmental stresses on children, in the hope of reducing their risk of substance abuse in years to come.

—ᴍ— Conclusion

Free to Grow eludes tidy definition, though its premise is simplicity itself: children are more likely to succeed in life if they grow up in homes and neighborhoods that are safe, stable, nurturing, and optimistic.

Most parents intuitively understand this—and want it for their children. Most social and political institutions understand it as well. This fundamental logic of Free to Grow breeds a contagious level of enthusiasm among its many partners—parents, neighborhood groups, police, social service agencies, and others drawn into the collaboration. It's certainly an easier sell than substance abuse education or treatment programs aimed at those already ensnared by alcohol, drugs, and tobacco. Efforts to safeguard the innocent young consistently draw broader public support than those aimed at helping already troubled teenagers or adults escape the consequences of bad choices. This popular—and political—bias toward the still undamaged young is not cynicism so much as human nature. It colors public policy well beyond the substance abuse field. In this context, Free to Grow's environmental interventions easily win converts. Things like better housing-code enforcement, neighborhood cleanup, traffic safety, and supervised after-school programs have obvious benefit to children, families, and communities, even if the stated long-term goal of Free to Grow—less drinking, drug taking, and smoking—remains elusive.

Implementing Free to Grow, however, isn't simple at all. Even in the relatively controlled environment of a demonstration project, Free to Grow quickly ballooned to encompass a dizzying array of interventions. Evidence of this abounded at the program's 2004 annual meeting, where phase-two grantees presented videos showing Free to Grow in action in their communities. One could pick out a common theme or technique here and there, but the larger impression was of a kaleidoscope of approaches, many of them unique to the conditions and the resources of a specific community. This decentralized program structure is consistent with Free to Grow's goal of empowering families and communities to effect *their* goals rather than imposing standards and priorities from the outside. The latter structure offers efficiency and a better shot at measurable results, especially in the context of a short-term, grant-funded experiment. Free to Grow seeks to plant the seeds for self-improvement in a way that continues to bear fruit after grantmakers withdraw.

That has proved to be the case in Owensboro, Kentucky, where the local Head Start program permanently incorporated the Free to Grow family assessment, in which caseworkers aggressively probe for drug addiction and other problems and direct parents to helpful community resources. The impact on this phase-one project six years after Free to Grow funding ended also is evident in continuing robust partnerships among agencies that previously worked on parallel—and sometimes competitive—tracks. Local leaders describe Free to Grow's role as similar to that of case managers for patients with complicated illnesses requiring the attention of many specialists working in concert. "You have all these systems in play: the police department does its thing, the schools do their thing, social services do their thing, but no one talks to the other agencies all working in the same neighborhood and sometimes with the same people," says Owensboro Police Lieutenant Ken Bennett. "With Free to Grow, we acted in a lot of ways like brokers for services from other city departments, like the housing-code enforcement or traffic enforcement."

In Kentucky and elsewhere, however, questions linger about the effectiveness of specific Free to Grow interventions, how best to deploy limited resources at the community level, and how to track impact. There's also discussion about whether Head Start is the best vehicle for such a wide-ranging social change project. The national evaluation is expected to shed light on many of these questions, but it's not designed to address the cost-benefit question—a key one for policymakers as well as budget-minded agency directors. At this writing, it's also unclear whether phase-two Head Start test sites will have the means to incorporate Free to Grow when Robert Wood Johnson Foundation funding runs out this year. Sarah Greene, the National Head Start Association's president and CEO, says the program is strapped for cash. Now budgeted at $6.1 billion, it has suffered a sharp decline since 2000 in appropriations for innovation, staff development, and other enhancements. Most Head Start agencies, according to Greene, are scrambling simply to sustain core services against rising costs. "It is a lot of work and it is costly, especially the family service part and intensive case management," Greene says of Free to Grow.

Free to Grow's costs go beyond dollars and cents. Local Head Start directors say it also exacts a human toll. This suggests yet another loose end as the demonstration project draws to a close: how to sustain the passion that everyone involved in Free to Grow—from national program leaders to local foot soldiers—says is necessary to sell the message of self-improvement, community building, and interagency cooperation. Carmen Nicholas, Head Start director in Palm Beach County, Florida, a phase-two Free to Grow site, says she has had to deal with burnout, especially among family service workers. Traditionally, these workers have come from the ranks of Head Start mothers. Nicholas and other directors say Free to Grow imposes quasi-professional duties on people who live in the same impoverished communities and may be friends, neighbors, or relatives of the very people they're obligated to question about drug use, domestic violence, and other family dysfunction. Beyond the awkwardness of uncovering these problems in a social peer is the sometimes long and frustrating road to alleviating them.

"It's hard work, and not all of these problems are quickly or easily solved, so my staff sometimes suffers heartache over failures," Nicholas says. "There's also an element of danger in questioning people about drug use. As director, I have had to do stress management in a number of ways, such as rotating people to lighter duties when I see them struggling with too many cases involving families with overwhelming needs." Finally, she must continually refresh her own passion for Free to Grow in order to sustain the vision in her staff of 300, who are spread among thirty preschool sites in Palm Beach County. "Free to Grow requires continuous training of workers," Nicholas says. "And some of them can't handle it or leave for better paying jobs, so there is constant staff turnover as well."

Head Start and Free to Grow aren't inseparable. Just as Free to Grow's community partners have found common ground, so might the program find another platform for its family- and community-strengthening strategies. The Justice Department's Weed and Seed program comes to mind, as do outreach projects of community development agencies. Indeed, the principles of collaboration and shared expertise that underpin Free to Grow ultimately lead back to the research world. The amazing performance of Foust Elementary School's fourth-graders provides a tantalizing illustration.

Half of the children who contributed to the rising test scores started out as Head Start preschoolers targeted by Owensboro's Free to Grow program since 1996. Interventions were guided by a body of research on risk and protective factors for substance abuse, and improved school performance was a hoped-for by-product. But what about the other children who show up each fall for kindergarten streetwise and very tough to settle down, in the words of Principal Jeff Gray.

This is where Gray's research mentors come into play, all from the field of early childhood education, but, like their counterparts in the substance abuse field, focused on risk factors for school failure among disadvantaged children and strategies for improving their chances of success. Gray put this research into practice by restructuring the system shortly after he took over as Foust's principal in 2000. "We had disruptive, disrespectful behavior, fighting, and so on," Gray says, "an unruly environment that interfered with everyone's ability to learn and intimidated many of the children."

Foust today has a strict disciplinary code that involves parents directly in goal setting and the enforcement of school standards. There's also a reward system for conduct, attendance, and academic achievement through which youngsters can earn "Foust dollars" to spend at the school store. Teachers are encouraged to expect performance as high as they would for their own children. "We read a book on all the excuses people make for not educating the poor: the testing materials are too hard, their parents don't care, they come to school with an empty belly," Gray says. "All these excuses were invalid, according to the research."

The restructuring activity at Foust was independent of Free to Grow. Where they intersected was Hager Preschool, a Head Start site on the Foust campus that had little interaction with Foust's kindergarten faculty before the inception of Free to Grow but now works in partnership on student assessments and curriculum planning. Even if the two camps arrived by different routes, laboring at the cutting edge of independent theories, they now share excitement over the achievements of children they collectively helped to rise above their circumstances.

And there's another buzz building—this time over a group of Foust third-graders who've been quietly working above grade level, so much so that they're poised to qualify for the school district's gifted and talented program. That would be another first for Foust—and for the children of Owensboro's West End.

Notes

1. Campbell, J. "Most Schools Performing Well but Some High Schools Need Work." *Owensboro Messenger-Inquirer,* Oct. 14, 2004, p. 1.
2. Catalano, R. S. "Free to Grow and Prevention Science." Presented at Free to Grow annual meeting, Maui, Hawaii, Nov. 10, 2004.
3. Hawkins, J. D., Catalano, R. F., and Miller, J. Y. "Risk and Protective Factors for Alcohol and Other Drug Problems in Adolescence and Early Adulthood: Implications for Substance Abuse Prevention." *Psychological Bulletin,* 1992, *112*(1), 64–105.
4. The Weed and Seed Strategy. Washington, D.C.: U.S. Department of Justice, Office of Justice Programs, Topical Publication Series NCJ #189318.

2

Improving Health in an Aging Society

Robin E. Mockenhaupt, Jane Isaacs Lowe,
and Geralyn Graf Magan[1]

Editors' Introduction

The aging of the American population represents a significant social challenge, one that will increase over the next fifty years. From a strictly economic perspective, as the debates over Social Security and Medicare illustrate, retirement and health care commitments must be financed for a growing number of retirees. More broadly, society needs to decide how to make sure the elderly stay healthy as long as possible, lead productive lives, and receive access to good medical care.

What will challenge health providers, policymakers, and families are the substantial inequalities that already exist within the elderly population and that promise to become even more pronounced in the future. Single, divorced, or widowed women as well as members of racial minorities—whose numbers will increase substantially—are especially vulnerable to debilitating chronic health problems, poverty, and unmet health and social needs as they age. As the older population grows, so will the number of vulnerable older people as well as the challenges involved in making sure that existing health, social services, housing, and environmental infrastructures have the capacity to serve them.

As Robin Mockenhaupt, Jane Isaacs Lowe, and Geralyn Graf Magan have written in this chapter, an aging population is also an opportunity. They have set the Foundation's work in aging into a context of what society needs to do to promote the health and well-being of older adults. The chapter presents five propositions about how people can age in a healthy way. For each proposition, the authors present the research supporting the proposition and then discuss the relevance of various Foundation-supported programs to the proposition. Using this format, they are able to review the successes and failures of a broad range of initiatives and to suggest future paths that the Foundation might take.

Robin Mockenhaupt is the deputy director of the Robert Wood Johnson Foundation's health group and has played a leadership role in developing initiatives to promote active living among the elderly. Jane Isaacs Lowe, a senior program officer and leader of the Foundation's team focused on improving services for vulnerable populations, has been involved in planning and monitoring many Foundation-funded programs to improve long-term care services for the elderly. Geralyn Graf Magan is a Maryland-based freelance writer specializing in issues affecting older people.

---

1. The authors would like to thank the following individuals who contributed to the development of various sections of the article: Jessica Siehl, Wendy Yallowitz, and Risa Lavizzo-Mourey.

—ɯ— **D**eclining birth rates, aging baby boomers, and a series of life-extending medical and public health advances have contributed to a demographic change—the aging of the American population—that promises to have wide-ranging implications for all aspects of society. As one example, 20 percent of Americans are expected to reach retirement age by 2030, compared with only 4 percent in 1900.[1] Not only are older adults[2] especially vulnerable to debilitating chronic health conditions and unmet medical and social needs, but the substantial social and economic inequalities that already exist within the elderly population promise to become more pronounced.

This demographic shift is widely viewed as a growing crisis. Ordinary citizens and policymakers alike often focus on fears that "greedy" older adults, who are wholly dependent on government programs, will deplete the nation's financial resources at the expense of younger generations. These fears tend to divert public attention from a deeper question: What quality of life do we as a nation want to provide for our older citizens? How we answer this question will affect the quality of life for all Americans in the decades ahead. It will also raise a number of challenges.

Over the past twenty-five years, the Robert Wood Johnson Foundation's efforts to address the health and supportive service needs of older adults have been driven by its concern that the acute care system has not been adequately meeting the complex needs of persons with disabilities and chronic illness. The Foundation has tried to improve systems of supportive services for older adults and persons with disabilities largely by making grants to improve home- and community-based services and to integrate health and long-term care services.

In the late 1990s, cognizant of the body of scientific evidence that behavioral strategies such as physical activity and tobacco cessation lead to improved health,[3] the Foundation made healthy communities and lifestyles a priority. This led to the development of programs for older adults that promoted physical activity, civic engagement, and elder-friendly communities. The Foundation has been able to use the program strategies at its disposal—including model development, convening, demonstrations, research, policy analysis, and communications—across the spectrum of aging from illness prevention and health promotion to civic engagement and long-term care.

The Foundation's efforts to improve the quality of life of older Americans can be viewed in the context of the efforts of the federal government and of other foundations. The Administration on Aging (part of the Department of Health and Human Services), which was created in 1965 by the Older Americans Act, makes grants to states for community planning and services programs, research, training, and demonstration projects in the field of aging. Federally funded Area Agencies on Aging fund nutrition, health promotion and disease prevention, in-home care, and other services that are provided locally to low-income seniors. The National Institute on Aging (part of the National Institutes of Health) was established in 1974 to provide leadership in, among other areas, aging research, training, and the dissemination of health information.

Many regional, community, and family foundations have made aging a grantmaking priority. Grantmakers in Aging, made up of foundations working in the field, provides support to its members and to those interested in expanding into this field. Among national philanthropies, the Hartford Foundation has focused on aging and health for the last twenty-five years, with a primary emphasis on training of physicians, nurses, and social workers. For more than twenty years, the Retirement Research Foundation has been funding service programs and research that address aging and retirement issues. More recently, Atlantic Philanthropies has given priority to workforce issues and civic engagement in its program on aging and health. California's Archstone Foundation funds only programs affecting older adults, such as those to reduce falls and to improve care toward the end of life.

As awareness about the aging of the American population spreads, so too does the sense that an increasing older population represents a challenge rather than an opportunity. Health experts familiar with the latest statistics issue dire warnings about the veritable plague of frailty, chronic illness, and dementia that threatens to affect most, if not all, members of a future aging cohort. Similarly, policymakers worry about the growing number of older people who will expect to receive Social Security checks each month, and those whose projected health care costs will overburden Medicare and Medicaid budgets.

Many concerns about the graying of America are warranted. After all, any population group that grows exponentially—whether that group comprises school-age children or eighty-five-year-olds—puts pressure on societal infrastructures. However, focusing only on the challenges has helped perpetuate the stereotype that old age has to be a time of disability and dependency. More important, it has diverted public attention from the fact that older people do continue to learn and grow after retirement, and that many continue to make significant contributions.

Drawing on the literature and on the Robert Wood Johnson Foundation's experience in the field, we have identified five propositions that can serve as a framework for discussions about aging and can help advocates, foundations, government agencies, and older consumers develop policies and programs that will promote the health and well-being of older adults.

Proposition 1: Older Age Does Not Have to Be Characterized by Disability and Dependency; Older People Can Make Meaningful Contributions to Their Community and to Society

The Rationale

Research suggests that while some older people face age-related declines, others continue to function as well as younger individuals; that many older people are healthy; and that age-related learning losses are often exaggerated and can be mitigated through intellectual stimulation and other strategies.[4, 5] Research also suggests that old age doesn't have to be a time of isolation. In fact, most older people cope well with the losses that come with aging, despite conventional wisdom suggesting that the elderly are an isolated group for whom widowhood, retirement, and the departure of grown children brings about an irreversible loss of social attachments and community ties.[6]

Many older people are already making significant contributions to society. One-third of adults over age fifty-five work outside the home, and many provide valuable assistance to family members by raising 3.8 million grandchildren and providing child care to an additional 6 million families.[7, 8] Older volunteers—from well-known people like President Jimmy Carter to ordinary citizens who donate their time in soup kitchens and schools—are demonstrating that engaged older adults can make a difference. And research shows that active individuals are more likely to remain physically and mentally fit and that those who are not regularly engaged with others are more likely to be in poor health.[9, 10]

Although many older people are involved in their communities, many more could be. Despite the potential for engaged older adults to make lasting contributions, the majority of seniors do not spend any significant time in service to their communities. The number of older volunteers has increased over the past few decades, but older Americans still volunteer less than any other age group. In part, this relative inactivity can be attributed to the fact that few communities have a formal infrastructure that effectively channels and manages the contributions of older people. Indeed, many public and private agencies and organizations across the country dedicate themselves to serving the elderly, but few agencies dedicate themselves to helping the elderly serve others.

While some older people find their fulfillment in volunteer activities, others remain active by staying on the job beyond normal retirement age. Eighty percent of baby boomers—those born between 1946 and 1964—say they plan to work at least part time during their retirement. About a quarter will work because they have to—they'll need the additional income to ensure their financial security. Thirty-five percent will work for the sheer pleasure of it.[11] The remaining percentage will structure paid employment to fit into their lifestyle and finances. This option may become less of a possibility once a worker reaches his or her late fifties. Despite the Age Discrimination in Employment Act, older workers throughout the nation continue to face both overt and subtle threats to their continued employment. Social Security and pension policies may force some older retirees to forego employment so they don't experience a reduction in their benefits. Employers may refuse to hire or promote older workers, encourage their early retirement, or target them if layoffs become necessary. Those who remain on the job may find themselves cut out of training opportunities or filling positions that seem to have fewer responsibilities with each passing year.

Policies and programs that encourage older people to volunteer or to remain in the workforce, though important, have been shown to be far more effective if they are combined with initiatives that encourage life-long learning among older people. Such learning opportunities could provide supplemental training to help older workers remain competitive in their own fields or start second careers after retirement. Learning that is aimed at self-enrichment could lead to more frequent and meaningful interaction among older people, and increased community engagement through volunteering. Fortunately, the availability of technology means that the homebound elderly don't have to miss out on these learning activities as long as they have a computer. Finally, programs that teach older people how to maintain a healthy lifestyle—for example, by sharing strategies that promote physical activity, a healthy diet, and early detection of disease—could help more Americans achieve a vigorous old age.[12]

Foundation-funded Programs

The Robert Wood Johnson Foundation has initiated several programs to help older people use their talents to address specific needs in local communities. The Experience Corps grew out of research conducted during the early 1990s by Public/Private Ventures—a nonprofit organization that works to improve the effectiveness of social policies—on the need to mobilize greater adult support for young people growing up in poverty. With funding from the Corporation for National Service and the Retirement Research Foundation, Public/Private Ventures and the late John Gardner led the team that launched the program in 1998, with five initial pilot sites. Civic Ventures was soon created to develop the Experience Corps into a national movement that would encourage older Americans to undertake public service in order to meet serious unmet community needs. Experience Corps members, most of whom give fifteen hours a week, work one-on-one with elementary schoolchildren who need intensive help learning to read. What began as a pilot program in five cities has grown—with funding from the Robert Wood Johnson Foundation, Atlantic Philanthropies, and many community funders—to include more than 1,500 volunteers in thirteen cities across the country. Such intergenerational mentoring programs have been highly effective in helping at-risk children avoid first-time drug use, improve school attendance, boost academic performance, and steer clear of violent behavior.[13] In addition to its benefits for students, the Experience Corps has also been shown to enhance the well-being of the volunteers. Physical, cognitive, and social activity increased in volunteers, suggesting the potential for Experience Corps and similar programs to improve health for an aging population while simultaneously improving educational outcomes for children.[14]

Similarly, Family Friends, an organization established in 1984 with funds from the National Council on the Aging, the Administration on Aging, and the Robert Wood Johnson Foundation, enlists older volunteers to help the families of children who have disabilities or suffer from chronic illnesses. It now operates at forty-three sites nationwide. Family Friends expanded this approach and now works with other groups, including the homeless and HIV-infected children, and at-risk children in poor rural communities. Adapting this model of intergenerational mentoring to teen pregnancy prevention, the Foundation funded Family Friends in 1998 to launch Generations Involved in Future Trust, or GIFT. It is the first initiative in the country to match older adults with young people with the idea of averting adolescent pregnancy.

Proposition 2: The Chances for Aging Successfully Can Be Improved by Physical and Mental Activity, Community Involvement, and the Use of Preventive Health Services

The Rationale

Summarizing eight years of research conducted under the MacArthur Foundation's Network on Successful Aging, John Rowe and Robert Kahn suggest that older people who are at low risk for disease and disease-related disability, and who have a high level of mental and physical functioning, are likely to weather old age better than those who don't enjoy these benefits.[15] The latter are at a greater risk of frailty and cognitive decline in their later years. Disability rates among older people fell during the 1980s, and a growing body of research shows that when people make certain lifestyle changes—like increasing their level of physical activity or taking advantage of preventive health care services—they reduce their risk of developing disabling conditions.[16] Communities can foster successful aging by ensuring that the design of the built environment and the services provided in communities promote physical activity and help older citizens live independent and productive lives.

Research studies have shown the powerful effect that regular physical activity can have on health and well-being. The Surgeon General of the United States reports that regular physical activity can reduce an individual's risk of developing coronary heart disease, hypertension, colon cancer, diabetes, depression, and anxiety, and that it can improve mood and enhance a person's ability to perform daily tasks.[17] Moreover, a regimen of physical activity can help increase levels of "good" cholesterol, improve balance, alleviate the aches and pains of arthritis, and save health care dollars.[18, 19, 20] In spite of these benefits, however, less than a third of older people follow the recommendations of the Centers for Disease Control and Prevention and the American College of Sports Medicine for a minimum of thirty minutes of moderate-intensity activity on most days of the week.[21] It remains to be seen how many older adults will follow the more recent guidelines from the Institute of Medicine on healthy eating and physical activity.

On the bright side, older people appear to be interested in increasing their physical activity, even though they haven't succeeded in doing so. A nationwide survey conducted by AARP found that 63 percent of people age fifty and older believe that exercise is the best thing they can do for their health. Nearly three-fourths of the 2,000 survey respondents said they are interested in learning how to exercise safely. Seventy-one percent said they want help staying motivated, and two-thirds expressed an interest in learning how to set realistic goals for physical activity.[22]

Many of the diseases that plague older adults could be prevented or delayed, or their seriousness could be diminished, through more widespread use of preventive health services. Yet fewer than half of Americans receive the preventive health services that are currently recommended by the federal Preventive Services Task Force, such as counseling for tobacco cessation, screening for vision impairments, and vaccinations against influenza and pneumococcal disease.[23] Depressive symptoms occur in approximately 15 percent of community residents 65 and older, yet depression often goes undiagnosed and untreated.[24, 25] In addition, some cognitive declines, such as memory loss, can be prevented through good nutrition, regular exercise, and continued engagement in certain leisure activities.[26]

Institutionalization can often be avoided if frail older people can find ways to stay in their own homes. But the desire of four out of five Americans to stay in their homes may be frustrated as long as American communities are designed only for young, able-bodied individuals. Suburban and rural communities—where 72 percent of the elderly now reside— often fail to provide the kinds of amenities that foster independent living.[27] For example, narrow doorways, long staircases, and second-floor master bedrooms—standard features of most residential dwellings—guarantee that even the most beloved family home will quickly become the homeowner's worst enemy when symptoms of frailty or disability appear. In addition, communities that fail to provide convenient public transportation, pedestrian-friendly streets, and shopping areas that are within walking distance of housing guarantee that older people who lose their driver's license will also lose their independence.

Elder-friendly communities anticipate and plan for the inevitable changes that occur as people age. They provide affordable housing designed for the entire life span and make it easy to walk or take a bus to needed services. At their best, they offer access to health care, clean, safe streets, good jobs and service opportunities, and a rich array of social and cultural activities.

Foundation-funded Programs

The Robert Wood Johnson Foundation has taken several steps to help older people increase their level of physical activity. A major Foundation initiative, Active for Life, is testing two promising strategies for getting large numbers of adults age fifty and older to incorporate physical activity into their daily lives and maintain an active lifestyle. The first strategy uses group-based problem-solving methods. The second emphasizes participation in individually selected physical activities, with telephone and e-mail follow-up. Nine grantees—they include aging, health, faith-based, recreation, and educational organizations—fund local organizations to carry out programs using one or the other of the strategies. An evaluation is assessing the process of reaching large numbers of midlife and older adults in their communities, and learning how organizations adapt program models. To support Active for Life, the Foundation funds a communications initiative, coordinated by AARP, aimed at helping communities promote physical activity, develop resources to help older residents become more active, and campaign for the removal of neighborhood barriers to physical activity.

Two related initiatives—Active Living by Design and Active Living Research—encourage community design, public policies, and communications strategies that promote physical activity. Under Active Living by Design, twenty-five community partnerships (consisting of a variety of organizations in public health and other disciplines, such as city planning, transportation, architecture, recreation, crime prevention, traffic safety and education, plus some key advocacy groups) are working to develop community design, public policies, and communications strategies that will increase physical activity. Several Active Living by Design sites focus on older adult populations in their efforts to make land use, public transit, nonmotorized travel, public spaces, parks, trails, and architectural practices friendlier to physical activity. Active Living Research funds research that examines relationships among natural and built environments, public and private policies, and personal levels of physical activity. It is establishing a transdisciplinary research base on the environmental and policy correlates of physical activity.

Promoting physical activity is also part of a Foundation-supported Senior Wellness Project, a service of Senior Services of Seattle/King County, a research-based health promotion and disease management program. The project was created to provide accessible, low-cost health promotion programs to older adults with chronic conditions. Its Health Enhancement Program helps older people create a health improvement plan in partnership with a registered nurse, a social worker, a primary care physician, and a volunteer mentor who provides one-on-one counseling and encouragement. To help participants carry out their plans, the Health Enhancement Program's wellness sites offer a daily hot lunch, exercise programs, nutrition and health education, interest groups and classes, volunteer opportunities, and assistance with transportation. The Senior Wellness Project has been shown to reduce hospitalization days and the use of medications and to improve the quality of life, physical activity, and functioning.[28]

The Vote and Vaccinate program was piloted in fifteen communities in the fall of 2004. Building on a Local Initiatives Funding Partners grant to SPARC, a community-based program that develops local strategies for increasing access to clinical preventive services in New England, Vote and Vaccinate provides immunizations to older adults at polling places on Election Day.

The AdvantAge Initiative, also funded by the Robert Wood Johnson Foundation, is developing a set of indicators to help communities assess how well they promote and facilitate independent living by older residents. Working initially in ten communities around the country, the AdvantAge Initiative surveyed older adults about how well their communities help them remain healthy, live independently, and lead productive and satisfying lives. In addition, to help other communities assess their ability to meet the needs of older residents, the initiative is providing assistance on collecting information, holding focus groups, and building coalitions. The initiative also profiled seventeen promising community efforts designed to maximize the potential for older residents to remain active, independent, and engaged. These include addressing the basic needs of older adults, such as housing and safety; encouraging physical activity and the use of preventive health services; promoting independence by improved caregiving and transportation; and advancing social and civic engagement, largely through volunteerism.

Proposition 3: Planning Early for Long-Term Care Can Give Older People the Security That They Will Be Able to Live Where They Choose as Long as Possible, Avoid Financial Ruin, and Have Health Care Decisions Made on the Basis of Their Own Preferences

The Rationale

Over the next several decades, the number of Americans needing long-term care will increase dramatically. How easily older adults and their families will be able to obtain this care will depend on their ability to navigate a complex service delivery system, find the right providers and the right coverage, and finance the care they will need. What makes understanding long-term care so difficult is that there is no single authoritative source of information or single point of entry. Long-term care is delivered in communities. It is not a unified system but, rather, a constellation of individual parts.

Many middle-aged and older adults do not know how or where to obtain impartial information that can help them plan for later-life care. It often takes a medical crisis to create a sense of urgency that forces older adults and their families to think about long-term care options, which, by then, are often limited and more expensive. The AdvantAge Initiative's 2003 national survey of adults age sixty-five and older found that 20 percent of older adults did not know whom to call for information about long-term care and supportive services.[29] Furthermore, those with physical limitations or poor health were the least likely to know how to get information. A recent AARP survey found that more than 60 percent of Americans age forty-five and older indicated some familiarity with long-term care services.[30] Most respondents in both surveys underestimated the cost of a nursing home (whose existence makes advance planning seem less critical) or they overestimated the cost of long-term care insurance (which makes them reluctant to buy a policy).[31] In addition, many seniors believe—incorrectly—that Medicare will pay for long-term care.

Foundation-funded Programs

Recognizing that most older adults want to remain in their homes and communities, in 2001 the Robert Wood Johnson Foundation funded the Community Partnerships for Older Adults, or CPOA, an eight-year $28 million initiative. The goal of this program is to build public-private community partnerships to improve long-term care and supportive services systems to meet the needs of older adults.

A key element of the program is the development of a model that provides reliable, up-to-date, and tailored information about long-term care services in the community. Each CPOA site is developing an information system that will allow older persons or their family members— especially recent immigrants and those who do not speak English, have limited health literacy, or confront other barriers to information and services—to make a single call to identify supportive services and determine eligibility. In nineteen locations across the country, CPOA grantees are educating members of their communities about long-term care and working to develop community-wide long-term care options. For example, through the Department of Aging and Adult Services, the San Francisco Partnership has launched SF-Get Care, a Web-based information and referral system that allows older adults and their families to locate in-home and community-based supportive services and other resources. In Hawaii, Maui Community Partnerships is using public access television to raise awareness about health care programs and services for older adults on the islands of Maui, Molokai, and Lanai.

Two other Foundation-funded programs help older adults learn more about long-term care: BenefitsCheckUp and Next Chapter (formerly Life Options). The BenefitsCheckUp program is an online service of the National Council on the Aging that helps people age fifty-five and older identify and apply for federal, state, and local programs. It provides information on prescription drugs, health coverage, payment of utility bills, volunteering, home-based services, and the like. Next Chapter, developed by Civic Ventures, is designed to help individuals nearing retirement answer the question, "What's next?" The program provides information on a range of topics—from opportunities for paid or volunteer employment to financial and long-term care planning—in libraries and community colleges.

Long-term care can be expensive. Home health care ranges from $12,000 to $50,000 a year, and assisted living, other residential alternatives, and nursing homes can cost upward of $80,000 a year. It should come as no surprise, therefore, that after paying for one year of long-term care, many older Americans find themselves impoverished and relying on Medicaid to cover the cost of their long-term care (as long as they qualify under the means test for the program in their home state).

Long-term care insurance is widely considered as a key component in guarding against the catastrophic costs associated with nursing homes, assisted living, and home health care. If purchased by enough people, long-term care insurance could also protect state Medicaid programs from carrying the entire long-term care financing burden of an aging population. Limited coverage and the high cost of long-term care insurance policies have, however, limited their appeal. Less than 10 percent of adults over sixty-five, and an even smaller percentage of those aged fifty-five to sixty-four, have purchased long-term care insurance.[32] The Health Insurance Portability and Accountability Act of 1996 took an important first step to making long-term care insurance more affordable by allowing purchasers of federally qualified long-term care insurance policies to deduct their premiums, up to a specified limit, on their federal income taxes.

Because of the high cost and the complexity of long-term care insurance, prospective buyers need objective information to help them decide whether this insurance is appropriate for them and, if so, which policy to buy. The Foundation has designed programs to help increase people's knowledge about both Medicare (which does not pay for long-term care but which enters into the consideration of long-term care options) and long-term care insurance (which does pay for long-term care). The Center for Medicare Education, funded in 1998 by the Robert Wood Johnson Foundation, has been an important resource for agencies and organizations that provide consumer education about the Medicare program. Likewise, the Medicare Rights Center, established in 1989 with funds from the Robert Wood Johnson Foundation and other foundations, provides free counseling services to people with issues concerning Medicare. Since its establishment, the Medicare Rights Center has helped more than a million people with Medicare-related issues through its counseling hotline, education sessions and materials, and technical assistance.

The Program to Promote Long-Term Care Insurance for the Elderly was funded between 1988 and 1998 to provide states with resources to organize partnerships of long-term care insurance companies and state Medicaid programs. The partnerships protect beneficiaries against losing everything if they need expensive long-term care. Instead, the costs are paid initially by a private insurance company and, if coverage runs out, by Medicaid. Even after support from the Robert Wood Johnson Foundation ended, public-private partnerships in California, Connecticut, Indiana, and New York continue to operate. By 2000, more than 95,000 partnership policies had been sold in these states, and more than 30 percent of the participants reported that they would not have purchased long-term care insurance without the partnership program. An independent evaluation found that the strict regulations governing the policies sold under the Program to Promote Long-Term Care Insurance for the Elderly resulted in higher-quality long-term care insurance coverage than was previously available in the states.[33]

Proposition 4: A More Efficient and Responsive Health and Supportive Care System Requires Better Coordination of Services and Information

The Rationale

Older people with complex health conditions often receive health and long-term care services from a number of providers, including primary care physicians, specialists, nurses, home health aides, social workers, and physical therapists. In fact, nearly a third of people with serious chronic conditions see four or more doctors at a time.[34] Many chronically ill people receive their care in a variety of settings: doctors' offices, hospitals, assisted-living locations, skilled nursing facilities, and their own homes. Many move from one setting to another in the course of a year.

This plethora of providers and settings makes care of the chronically ill extremely difficult. Health care providers and informal caregivers find it challenging, and sometimes impossible, to ensure that an individual's long-term care plan follows him or her from one setting to the next. Lack of communication among an individual's health care professionals can exacerbate the difficulty that patients encounter when they make these transitions. Moreover, older adults living in the community may not know what services they need or how to find the ones they want. Those who require services from different agencies may find it overwhelming to keep straight the programs' varied eligibility requirements and their unique sets of service providers and financing systems. These challenges, taken together, often keep chronically ill older people from receiving a full range of home- and community-based services.

Navigating the maze of programs and services can be hard for both rich and poor. A low-income person, for example, may qualify for publicly funded long-term care services but may have no idea that such services are available or how to learn about them. Persons with higher incomes may correctly assume that they can't take advantage of public services but may have little idea about how to find the ones they need, at an affordable price, in the private sector.[35]

Foundation-funded Programs

To help improve the coordination of services for older people living in the community, the Foundation has supported the development of programs that sought to integrate housing, health, and social services by placing these services in a single location or by integrating the way they were financed. In the mid-1980s, several Foundation programs integrated social services for frail elders into federally subsidized housing for seniors. This concept was expanded to include incorporating social services into housing in naturally occurring retirement communities—housing developments, apartment buildings, and neighborhoods in which residents had aged in place and that had high concentrations of older people. The Coming Home program, for example, developed a model of affordable assisted living that combined housing and social services for older adults in small towns and rural areas in ten states.

In addition, the Foundation supported several programs that integrated Medicare and Medicaid financing in order to create a seamless system of health and social services integration for frail older adults. The Program of All-Inclusive Care for the Elderly, or PACE, provides team-managed care that integrates acute and long-term health services in both inpatient and outpatient settings for elderly people. "Social health maintenance organizations," developed in the 1980s, were viewed as a way of improving care for frail elderly people by combining managed care and expanded home- and community-based services. The Medicare/Medicaid Integration Program is a fourteen-state demonstration that tests the operation and design of delivery systems that integrated long-term and acute care services under combined Medicare and Medicaid capitation payments for elderly patients.

In 1992, as the Robert Wood Johnson Foundation developed a more formal funding strategy for its grantmaking in chronic illness care, it applied lessons from these earlier programs to a new program, Building Health

Systems for People with Chronic Illnesses. This program funded demonstration projects designed to overcome the fragmentation, financing barriers, and episodic care that characterized existing systems of care for older adults, people with physical and mental disabilities, and children with special needs. Six of the thirty-two demonstration projects focused on frail older adults. These projects sought to link acute and long-term care services for older adults who might otherwise be in nursing homes but were residing in their own homes or in personal care homes.

Community Partnerships for Older Adults, referred to earlier, also supports efforts to develop coordinated service systems. For example, the Atlanta Community Partnerships program, Aging Atlanta, has developed Care Options, an online care coordination system that will allow for electronic updates of changes in a client's needs.

Proposition 5: Successful Aging Will Require a More Highly Trained and Qualified Workforce of Paid and Unpaid Caregivers

The Rationale

Most of the country's long-term care services are dispensed by informal caregivers such as family members and close friends in individual homes. As more long-term care is provided at home and in the community rather than through institutions, reliance on family and informal caregivers will continue to grow. Providing this support is no small feat, given the sheer numbers of relatives and friends who care for older people. Nearly one out of every four households—about 22 million—is involved in caring for a person aged fifty and older, while 5 million households care for an older person with dementia.[36] Sixty percent of these caregivers either work or have worked while providing care, and have had to make some adjustments to their work life, from reporting late to work to giving up work entirely. Although this arrangement saves the nation billions of dollars a year, informal caregiving does not come without a price. Nearly a third of those caring for persons age sixty-five and older describe their own physical health as fair to poor. As many as 11 million informal caregivers may suffer from the symptoms of depression.[37]

Informal caregivers lack information, training, and support. The need to strengthen and sustain families in their caregiving role is becoming a key issue in our society. Caregivers who receive support, such as education and skills training, counseling, and respite care for themselves and coordinated services for their care recipient, tend to have better health than those who do not receive such support. Caregivers who take their loved one to an adult day care center, for example, experience less stress and better psychological well-being than those who don't.

Beyond nonpaid caregiving, a trained and qualified paid workforce is essential to providing quality care. Yet there is a shortage of frontline workers, such as home health aides, companions, nursing assistants, and community health workers, that threatens to compromise the ability of health care systems to respond to the growing need for personal care among older adults. Although the number of elders who need help with daily activities will more than double, to 11 million from 5 million by 2050, the supply of elder-care workers is expected to decline during the same period.[38]

Annual staff turnover rates of 45 percent for nursing homes and 10 percent for home health programs are a big part of the problem. High turnover rates can result in poor quality and unsafe care for patients, higher levels of stress for workers who remain in understaffed workplaces, and increased pressure on family members who often must fill in the care gaps. They also cost health care providers millions of dollars in recruitment, training, and lost productivity.

High turnover rates are due, in part, to the low pay, difficult working conditions, and high demands on those caring for elderly people. The typical paraprofessional is a single mother with a high school degree or less, who earns between $6.50 and $8.50 an hour. Many of these people hold two jobs, and most live below the federal poverty level.[39] Few receive employer-paid health insurance, and supportive supervision is rare. On top of this, inadequate training leaves most paraprofessionals ill-prepared to provide the level of care required by the chronically ill patient. Medicare requires that nursing home assistants receive only seventy-five hours of training, with only sixteen hours of that training devoted to supervised, hands-on work. Some states set additional standards for training, but the rigorousness of these training standards varies widely.

Foundation-funded Programs

It would be difficult to overstate the importance of neighborhood volunteers in supporting caregivers and providing services to older people living in the community. Neighbors and other community members who befriend chronically ill elderly people and their caregivers help lessen the isolation that older people experience, offer vital services that help them remain in their communities, provide respite for family members providing care, and save health care dollars by reducing the need for paid service providers. The Faith in Action program, initially funded in 1992, brings together volunteers of many faiths to provide assistance with daily activities to those with long-term health needs. It has provided seed grants to more than a thousand interfaith coalitions in communities across the United States.

From 1992 to 2001, the Foundation supported the development and expansion of Partners in Caregiving, a program that allows older adults with dementia or chronic illness (or both) to continue living at home yet receive the care they need in adult day centers. These centers, in communities in thirteen states, provide health, social, and support services for adults with impaired physical, mental, and social abilities. At the same time, they allow family caregivers a much-needed respite, and also allow them to continue working if they need to earn a living. In 2000, a Foundation-funded study of adult day services documented the need for more centers.

Through its Cash & Counseling program, the Foundation has given home-bound disabled people the option of choosing whom to pay for their home care. Many have decided to pay family members or other informal caregivers who otherwise would have had to volunteer their time or not be able to do it at all. The program began as a two-state demonstration and was expanded to eleven states in 2004. As a result of this program, the federal Centers for Medicare & Medicaid Services now supports state Medicaid demonstrations to develop consumer-directed options for beneficiaries who receive long-term care.

Another program that focused on advancing consumer choice in long-term care was Independent Choices. It was designed to complement the Cash & Counseling program by supporting smaller-scale demonstration projects and research. Individual projects were chosen to address diverse populations and to test alternative approaches to the cash option for empowering consumers of long-term care. For example, several research projects explored older adult preferences for consumer-directed care, and the demonstration projects ranged from expanding available options for those who receive Medicaid long-term home care services to developing emergency backup services for people with disabilities.

Recent Foundation efforts have focused on finding ways to increase the number and the expertise of paraprofessional caregivers. The Better Jobs, Better Care program, jointly funded by the Robert Wood Johnson Foundation and Atlantic Philanthropies, is designed to create changes in policy and practice through demonstration and research grants that will lead to the recruitment and retention of high-quality direct care workers in both nursing homes and home and community settings. During 2003, five state-based coalitions consisting of providers, workers, and consumers were awarded grants of up to $1.4 million each to strengthen practices and policies in order to attract and retain high-quality paraprofessionals. The demonstration project in North Carolina, for example, aims at developing a special licensure designation for home care agencies and for residential and nursing facilities. The project in Pennsylvania is establishing a statewide nonprofit entity to promote policies, such as wage increases, mentoring, and the adoption of uniform training standards across all long-term care settings, that can improve the quality of care and retention of workers. In addition, Better Jobs, Better Care awarded grants of up to $500,000 to eight university-based researchers and nonprofit organizations to examine programs and policies thought to be successful in recruiting and retaining high-quality long-term care workers.

—ⱱ— **Future Directions**

It is evident that the time has come to change the images, stereotypes, perceptions, and the language around aging and to develop new approaches to healthy aging. At present, images tend toward two extremes—the eighty-year-old running the marathon or the eighty-year-old tied to a chair in a nursing home. The reality is that aging, unlike child development, is incredibly variable and does not meet an expected set of milestones. It is the lack of predictability in aging that results in many different pathways from midlife to the end of life. The continuum of aging from well to chronically ill to frail is not linear, and older adults frequently move among these categories. The propositions presented in this chapter can serve as guideposts for transforming how aging is viewed, for supporting the active participation and contributions of older adults in society, and for creating services that support and empower frail older adults and their families. Individuals, professionals serving older people, organizations, and society need to examine their stereotypes and create new images that support meaningful and productive living in the second half of life.

The twenty-first century will continue to see the rapid growth of an aging population. The number of people living beyond eighty-five will continue to increase. As a result, there are likely to be more people in their fifties and sixties who have surviving older relatives and therefore increased responsibilities for their care. Women will continue to become the majority of the oldest old, and they will face significant health, social, and economic problems, including living alone, increasing needs for supportive services, and higher levels of poverty. Finally, as illustrated in the report, *A Tale of Two Older Americas: Community Opportunities and Challenges,* the "fortunate majority" of older adults are thriving and experiencing good health, strong social connections, and adequate resources, while the "frail fraction" are in poor health and with inadequate financial security.[40] These two groups can reside in separate neighborhoods or live within the same apartment building. It is this second group—those with incomes below 200 percent of the poverty level, with less than a high school education, and with poor health status and limitations in daily activities—that needs attention. Within the frail population are many minorities and immigrant groups, reflecting the increased diversity in the older adult population. The challenge for those concerned with healthy aging is to develop a set of programs and interventions that will reach the increasingly heterogeneous older adult population, and especially the frail fraction.

Research has shown that healthy aging results from physical activity (which can be done by almost all adults, even the frail), mental activity, preventive care, connecting with others, engaging in meaningful activities, and knowing where and how to get supportive services. There is a need to translate research findings into practices that are accessible to older adults regardless of income, living situation, or culture. Although few organizations and communities are currently equipped to provide them, services can and should be designed to meet the needs of a culturally, linguistically, and educationally diverse older population.

By increasing both paid and volunteer opportunities for service, later life could be a time when older people, both the fortunate majority and the frail fraction, make their most lasting impact on their families, their places of work, and their communities. The Older Americans Act of 1965 helped raise the public's awareness of aging issues and made possible a range of programs, organized by the Administration on Aging, that continue to offer important services and opportunities. A similar national policy on the employment of older workers and an initiative on volunteerism would increase understanding of the importance of providing older people with options for meaningful activities. Individual organizations, both public and private, are already playing an important role in promoting opportunities for paid work and volunteerism among the elderly, but they can't do it alone. To be most successful, such a promotional effort should be rooted in a strong national organization that could gain the attention of both the public and private sectors.

Elderhostel and programs like it have been extremely successful in demonstrating that one is never too old to learn new things or enjoy new adventures. These programs should be replicated and expanded so that opportunities for growth and intellectual stimulation will be widely available to all older people, regardless of income or ability to travel. Because of their unique status within the senior community, senior centers may be able to play a central role in this effort. In addition, technology, which is bringing learning opportunities to homebound and other older people, should be expanded. Colleges, universities, and other learning institutions should be encouraged to develop learning materials that can be shared with older adults through the Internet.

Traditionally, health, housing, and social services have been divided into distinct professional and service sectors. Yet as people age, this separation does not make sense; health, housing, and services ought to become indistinguishable. For example, many older adults with limited financial resources live in an aging housing stock. It is often difficult to differentiate a housing crisis (for instance, no railings in the bathtub) from a health crisis (such as a broken hip). Partnerships of public and private funders, housing developers, the aging services network, and government need to work together to expand and refine community models that integrate or coordinate health, housing, and other services. These integrated systems of support save money, improve health outcomes, and decrease the frustration, confusion, and stress among older people and their caregivers. A great deal can be learned from emerging models of supportive housing such as shared housing arrangements, senior housing, intergenerational housing, and new forms of assisted living.

Finally, strong partnerships should be developed to create communities for all ages. What older adults want in their communities—affordable housing, safe neighborhoods, transportation, recreation spaces, access to work or volunteer activities—is what families and younger adults want as well. These partnerships may involve unlikely partners, such as transportation, land use, health, recreation, and children's organizations. The challenge is combining the interests of these divergent community groups to reach common goals. This can happen through increased dialogue between organizations and individuals about important community and societal values.

The five propositions on aging can become a reality so that all older adults, their families, and their neighbors can support and safeguard their health and their independence.

Appendix: Examples of Major Robert Wood Johnson Foundation Programs on Aging

Building of Organizational and Community Capacity

AdvantAge Initiative (1999–2001, $200,000) is a community-building effort focused on creating elder-friendly, or "AdvantAged," communities that are prepared to meet the needs of older adults. This initiative began as a multifoundation collaborative to create benchmarks for elder-friendly communities. Using these benchmarks, ten communities across the United States tested and developed strategies to address the needs of their older adults.

Building Health Systems for People with Chronic Illness (1992–2002, $13 million) encompassed a broad range of initiatives covering the medical, mental health, and supportive services needs of frail elders, people with disabilities, children with special needs, and people with severe mental illness. Each project used a broadly inclusive definition of health and the health system, sought to reduce fragmentation in service delivery and financing, and included consumer-directed principles in the design and implementation of health and supportive services systems.

Community Partnerships for Older Adults (2000–2010, $26 million) fosters community partnerships to improve long-term care and supportive services to meet the current and future needs of older adults. This program provides funds for both development and implementation grants for thirty community grantees (www.partnershipsforolderadults.org/).

On Lok Senior Health Services (1983–1987, $649,930) began as a neighborhood-based alternative to nursing home care. It provided mobile support services in the home as well as centralized off-site care at an adult day health care center, and created a fully integrated model of acute and long-term care for low-income seniors that blends Medicare and Medicaid financing.

Program of All-Inclusive Care for the Elderly (PACE) (1993–1996, $1.2 million) was a replication of On Lok. PACE programs provided and coordinated all needed preventive, primary, acute, and long-term care services so that older individuals could continue living in the community.

Program for Health-Impaired Elderly (1979–1986, $7.7 million) was developed to address an intrinsic defect in the provision of services to the elderly—the absence of mechanisms or strategies to coordinate and prioritize services needed for health-impaired elderly people residing in the community.

Teaching Nursing Home Program (1981–1987, $6.7 million) was designed to improve the quality of nursing home care and the clinical training of nurses by linking nursing schools with nursing homes. Grants were made to eleven university nursing schools.

Civic Engagement and Physical Activity

Active for Life (2001–2007, $17 million) is a national program to encourage adults fifty and older to increase their activity levels. The program replicates and expands models demonstrated to be effective in increasing levels of physical activity.

Active Living by Design (2001–2008, $15.5 million) is a national program that attempts to harness community design and livable community initiatives as a vehicle for making communities more activity-friendly.

Active Living Research (2000–2007, $12.5 million) supports research to identify environmental factors and policies that influence physical activity. Findings from this research are used to help inform policy, the design of the built environment, and other factors to promote active living.

Experience Corps (2001–2006, $6.8 million) is an intergenerational project testing a well-developed model for making matches between children and older adults in public schools.

Health Enhancement Program (1999–2002, $194,000) was a participant-directed program for seniors to change health behavior, supported by a nurse–social worker–peer health mentor team and complemented by courses in exercise and self-management of chronic conditions. The program was offered to seniors in low-income, multi-ethnic public housing facilities and an African American senior center.

Expansion of a Senior Wellness Program (2001–2003, $750,000) entailed expansion of the Health Enhancement Program. This program integrated three critical elements of health enhancement for older adults—self-management of chronic disease, physical activity, and social support—in a variety of settings.

Improving Physical Activity Levels of Mid-Life and Older Adults (2001–2005, $4.3 million) has been a national program housed at AARP that aims at replicating programs shown to be effective in encouraging adults fifty and older to increase their levels of physical activity.

National Blueprint on Physical Activity Among Adults Age 50 and Older (2001–2005, $670,000) was an effort led by six partner organizations (AARP, American College of Sports Medicine, American Geriatrics Society, the Centers for Disease Control and Prevention, National Institute on Aging, and the Robert Wood Johnson Foundation) to create a national framework for planning, collaborative action, and social change among organizations and agencies involved in physical activity, aging, or both.

Education and Advocacy

Center for Medicare Education (1998–2002, $5.4 million) has been a resource for public agencies and private organizations that provide consumer education about the Medicare program and its health plan options. The center is part of the Institute for the Future of Aging Services, a policy research institute within the American Association of Homes and Services for the Aging.

Creation of a Counseling and Assistance Program for People with Medicare 2002–2003, $100,000) was initiated by the Medicare Rights Center, a Medicare counseling and assistance system that helps New Yorkers with Medicare obtain the Medicare benefits and health care services they need quickly and easily.

Financing and Policy

Cash & Counseling (1995–2008, $12 million) provides funding for elderly and disabled people that enables them to choose the people who provide their care and to pay them directly.

Independent Choices (1995–2000, $3.3 million) was designed to complement the Cash & Counseling program by providing funding for small-scale demonstrations and research designed to develop and test other approaches to empower consumers of long-term care.

The Medicare/Medicaid Integration Program (1996–2006, $4.5 million) addresses the financing and policy changes necessary to integrate these two funding streams for disabled older adults. This demonstration program tests the operation and design of delivery systems that integrate long-term and acute care services under combined Medicare and Medicaid capitation payments for elderly patients in fourteen states.

Program to Promote Long-Term Care Insurance for the Elderly (1988–1998, $12 million) was created to provide states with resources to plan and implement private-public partnerships that would join private, long-term care insurance with Medicaid to offer high-quality insurance protection against impoverishment from the costs of long-term care. Eight states received initial planning grants and four received implementation grants.

Promoting Long-Term Care Policy Development and Debate (2001–2004, $3.4 million) was created to renew interest in financing and policy change by establishing a broader understanding of the financing of long-term care, developing a range of potential policy solutions, and analyzing the costs of the newly created proposals. Based at Georgetown University, the program was seeking different answers to the question of how to cope with long-term care and its service needs.

Service Credit Banking Program for the Elderly (1986–1990, $1.1 million) was designed to assist consortia of community groups to expand the concept of service credit banking, under which elderly individuals volunteered to provide services to other elderly people and, in return, received credits that were redeemed for similar services at a later point.

Service Credit Banking in Managed Care (1994–1999, $600,000) provided technical assistance and information for the replication of service credit banking programs and sought to demonstrate the feasibility of establishing a service credit banking project within a managed care organization.

Social Health Maintenance Organization (1983–1994, $1 million) was created to reduce the cost and improve the quality of care for the elderly. This was to be achieved by combining the services of the fragmented health and long-term care systems into a single social HMO entity. (This was before the passage of legislation allowing for the development of Medicare managed care organizations.)

State Solutions (2001–2006, $4 million) has been a national program working to increase enrollment in and access to the Medicare savings programs, which are directed to low-income older people. State Solutions provides technical assistance and direction to grant recipients and disseminates information about innovative and promising practices throughout the nation.

Housing with Services

Coming Home: Integrated Systems of Care for the Rural Elderly (1992–2005, $13 million) has had as its goal the development of affordable assisted living as an integral part of the long-term care system for low-income elders in rural areas. Coming Home operates through a revolving loan fund managed by the NCB Development Corporation, which acts as a fiscal and technical assistance intermediary to organize community partners, make loans and grants for site analyses and predevelopment costs, and help arrange for long-term financing through NCB or other commercial lenders.

The Green House Model (2002–2006, $1 million) has sought to create an environment in which the frail elderly could receive medical assistance without being required to live in a large institution. Each Green House facility is designed to be a home for eight to ten people. Though technically licensed as a health care facility and not as private housing, this model expands the boundaries of what can be considered supportive housing.

Supportive Services Program for Older Persons (1985–1991, $8.5 million) was designed to promote the expansion of nontraditional health and heath-related services to the elderly, including services such as respite care, housekeeping, home repair, and transportation. This led to a shift in policy that allowed for the inclusion of services in Section 202 subsidized housing.

Supportive Services in Senior Housing (1987–1995, $3 million) sought innovative approaches to financing and delivering supportive services to people who lived in subsidized housing projects for the elderly.

Informal and Formal Caregiving

Better Jobs, Better Care (2002–2006, $8 million) is a research and demonstration program created to improve the recruitment and retention of quality nursing assistants, home health aides, and personal care attendants who care for elderly people with chronic diseases or disabilities. It is funded by the Robert Wood Johnson Foundation and Atlantic Philanthropies.

Faith in Action (Phase I, 1992–1999, $36 million; Phase II, 1999–2007, $50.5 million) has the primary goal of helping communities care for the growing number of people with chronic illness and disability who wish to remain in their own homes but need some assistance with daily activities. It makes grants to local interfaith groups that provide volunteers to care for their neighbors with long-term health needs.

Family Friends (1985–1991, $3.7 million) was a demonstration program based on a successful pilot project in Washington, D.C., conducted by the National Council on the Aging, with Foundation support. The program was designed to match older volunteers (age fifty-five and older) with chronically ill or disabled children and their families. Volunteers worked with children and their families in the families' homes. The goal of the program was to demonstrate the feasibility, value, and sustainability of the Family Friends model in different geographical locations under different types of organizational sponsorship.

Partners in Caregiving: The Dementia Services Program (1992–2001, $4.2 million) built on the lessons from an earlier adult day care program, the Dementia Care and Respite Services Program, which the Foundation funded between 1988 and 1992. In expanding the scope of that earlier program to all fifty states and the District of Columbia, Partners in Caregiving demonstrated that the adult day care model could be used for older adults with other chronic illnesses.

Notes

1. Siegel, J. *Aging into the 21st Century.* Washington, D.C.: Administration on Aging, U.S. Department of Health and Human Services, 1996. Available at (http://www.aoa.gov/prof/Statistics/future_growth/aging21/aging_21.asp).

2. The terms "older adult," "older people," "elder," and "elderly" are used throughout this chapter. Although many programs and services have age restrictions, there are no commonly accepted conventions for age-related terminology. "Older adult" is a generic term that is used most often in this chapter. However, if programs or services are specifically designed for the old or very old (seventy-five years or older), the term "elderly" may be used.

3. McGinnis, J. M., and Foege, W. H. "Actual Causes of Death." *Journal of the American Medical Association,* 1993, *270*(18), 2207–2212.

4. Powell, D. H. *The Nine Myths of Aging: Maximizing the Quality of Later Life.* New York: Freeman, 1998.

5. Rowe, J. W., and Kahn, R. L. *Successful Aging.* New York: Pantheon Books, 1998.

6. Berkman, L. F. "The Role of Social Relations in Health Promotion." *Psychosomatic Medicine,* 1995, *57*(3), 245–254.

7. Kinsella, K., and Gist, Y. J. *Older Workers, Retirement and Pensions: A Comparative Chartbook.* Washington, D.C.: U.S. Department of Commerce, 1995.

8. Bryson, K., and Casper, L. M. "Coresident Grandparents and Grandchildren." *Current Population Reports.* Washington, D.C.: U.S. Census Bureau, 1999.

9. Hall, M., and Havens, B. *The Effect of Social Isolation and Loneliness on the Health of Older Women.* Winnipeg, Manitoba, Canada: Prairie Women's Health Centre of Excellence, 1999.

10. Ham, B. "Social Isolation Leaves Elderly at Risk for Heart Trouble." Health Behavior News Service, Washington, D.C.: Center for the Advancement of Health. Accessed Nov. 28, 2002 from (http://www.hbns.org/news/lonely12-10-02.cfm).

11. AARP. *Baby Boomers Envision Their Retirement: An AARP Segmentation Analysis.* Washington, D.C.: AARP, 1999. Available from (www.aarp.org).

12. Wolff, L. "Lifelong Learning for the Third Age." Paper based on a meeting on Inter-Regional Consultation on Aging of the Population, hosted by the Inter-American Development Bank, June 2000. Available at (http://www.iadb.org/sds/doc/Edu&Tech20.pdf).

13. Tierney, J. P., and Grossman, J. B. *Making a Difference: An Impact Study of Big Brothers and Big Sisters.* Philadelphia, Pa.: Public/Private Ventures, 1995.

14. Fried, L., et al. "A Social Model for Health Promotion for an Aging Population: Initial Evidence on the Experience Corps Model." *Journal of Urban Health,* 2004, *81,* 64–78.

15. Rowe, J. W., and Kahn, R. L. *Successful Aging.* New York: Pantheon Books, 1998.

16. Kinsella, K., and Velkoff, V. A. *An Aging World: 2001.* Washington, D.C.: National Institute on Aging and the U.S. Census Bureau, 2002.

17. National Center for Chronic Disease Prevention and Health Promotion. *Physical Activity and Health: A Report of the Surgeon General.* Atlanta, Ga.: U.S. Department of Health and Human Services, Centers for Disease Control and Prevention, 1996.

18. National Institutes of Health. *Physical Activity and Cardiovascular Health.* NIH Consensus Statement, *13*(3). Bethesda, Md.: NIH, 1995.

19. Kovar, P. A., Allegrate, J. P., MacKenzie, C. R., Peterson, M. G., Gutin, B., and Charlson, M. E. "Supervised Fitness Walking in Patients with Osteoarthritis of the Knee: A Randomized Controlled Study." *Annals of Internal Medicine,* 1992, *116*(7), 529–534.

20. Yaffe, K., Barnes, D., Kevitt, M., Lui, L., and Covinsky, K. "A Prospective Study of Physical Activity and Cognitive Decline in Elderly Women: Women Who Walk." *Archives of Internal Medicine,* 2001, *161*(14), 1703–1708.

21. Centers for Disease Control and Prevention. *Promoting Active Lifestyles Among Older Adults.* Atlanta, Ga.: CDC, 2002.

22. Magan, G. G. "Communicating with the 50+ Audience About Physical Activity Issues." Paper presented in preparation for meeting on the Role of the Consumer in Promoting Physical Activity Through Health Care Settings, 2002, Washington, D.C.

23. Coffield, A., Maciosek, M. V., McGinnis, J. M., Harris, J. R., Caldwell, M. B., Teutsch, S. M., Atkins, D., Richland, J. H., and Haddix, A. "Priorities Among Recommended Preventive Services." *American Journal of Preventive Medicine,* 2001, *21*(1), 1–9.

24. National Institutes of Health. *Consensus Development Panel on Depression in Late Life, 9*(3), 1–27. NIH Consensus Statement. Bethesda, Md.: NIH, 1991.

25. U.S. Department of Health and Human Services. *Mental Health: A Report of the Surgeon General.* Washington, D.C.: Author, 2000.

26. Scarmeas, N., Levy, G., Tang, M-X, Manly, J., Stern, Y., et al. "Influence of Leisure Activity on the Incidence of Alzheimer's Disease." *Neurology,* 2001, *57,* 2, 2236–2242.

27. O'Dell, J. "Elderly Housing and Affordability Issues for the 21st Century." Testimony of Jane O'Dell, AARP Board of Directors, before the Housing and Community Opportunity Subcommittee of the House Financial Services Committee, July 17, 2001.

28. "The Robert Wood Johnson Foundation Supports the Health Enhancement Program." *Access: A Guide to Resources,* August 2001. Seattle, Wash.: Senior Services of Seattle/King County.

29. Feldman, P. H., et al. *A Tale of Two Older Americas: Community Opportunities and Challenges.* New York: Center for Home Care Policy and Research, 2004.

30. *The Costs of Long-Term Care: Perceptions Versus Reality.* Washington, D.C.: AARP, 2001.

31. National Council on the Aging. "Americans Look to Employers and Government for Help with Long-Term Care." Press Release, March 23, 1999. Available at ⟨http://www.ncoa.org/content.cfm?sectionID=105&detail=48⟩.

32. Senate Committee on Aging. Testimony on Long Term Care, "Baby Boom Generation Increases Challenge of Financing Needed Services," March 27, 2001.

33. Crum, R. "Program to Promote Long Term Care Insurance for the Elderly, National Program Report." The Robert Wood Johnson Foundation, Nov. 2003. Available at ⟨http://www.rwjf.org/reports/npreports/elderlye.htm⟩.

34. Partnership for Solutions. *Chronic Conditions: Public Perceptions About Health Care Access and Services.* Baltimore, Md.: Partnership for Solutions, 2002.

35. Reinhard, S. C., and Scala, M. A. *Navigating the Long-Term Care Maze: New Approaches to Information and Assistance in Three States.* Washington, D.C.: AARP Public Policy Institute, 2001.

36. Family Caregiver Alliance. *Fact Sheet: Selected Caregiver Statistics.* San Francisco: FCA, 2001.

37. Gray, L. *Caregiver Depression: A Growing Mental Health Concern.* San Francisco: Family Caregiver Alliance, 2003.

38. Brown, N. P. "A Crisis in Caregiving: Longer-Range Solutions for Long-Term Care." *Harvard Magazine,* Jan.-Feb. 2002, *104*(3).

39. National Clearinghouse on Direct Care Workforce. "Who Are the Direct Care Workers?" 2004. (http://www.paraprofessional.org/publications/NCDCW_0904_Fact_Sheetfinal.pdf).

40. Feldman, P. H., et al. *A Tale of Two Older Americas: Community Opportunities and Challenges.* New York: Center for Home Care Policy and Research, 2004.

From the Foundation's
Targeted Portfolio

The Robert Wood Johnson Foundation's Efforts to Cover the Uninsured

Robert Rosenblatt

Editors' Introduction

The United States is the only developed country without universal access to health insurance, and today forty-five million Americans—many of them minorities or poor people—lack coverage for basic health care. It is now well established that people without health insurance receive less medical care, even needed medical care, and are in poorer health than people who have coverage. It is also known that the lack of health insurance has led to the overuse of hospital emergency rooms—an expensive last resort—and, because people are sicker when they finally decide to get care, has led to unnecessarily high-cost hospitalizations and treatment.

This chapter, by Robert Rosenblatt, a former *Los Angeles Times* correspondent and currently a freelance writer specializing in health care issues, traces the Foundation's thirty-plus years of effort to increase Americans' access to health insurance. Rosenblatt observes that the Foundation has used three fundamentally distinct but not necessarily mutually exclusive strategies in addressing this enduring problem. It has supported efforts to bring about fundamental overhaul of the system (though it has never agreed on a single approach to doing so). It has worked to expand insurance coverage incrementally. And it has funded research to provide a better understanding of the dynamics of the system and an empirical basis for policy decisions.

The story of the Foundation's efforts to expand insurance coverage does not have a happy ending at this point: the percentage of uninsured Americans remains approximately the same in 2005 as it was thirty years ago. Nonetheless, the Foundation's commitment to expanding health insurance coverage is unwavering, and this chapter places the Foundation's work into a perspective that provokes thoughts about the next steps.

—m— There is a doctor in California's San Fernando Valley who will see patients the same day they call for an appointment. This doctor—let's call him David Dawson—will talk at some length about a patient's medical history and then perform an examination. The price is $85, payable in cash or by credit card. Many of Dr. Dawson's patients have medical insurance, through jobs in Los Angeles' high-tech companies or the entertainment industry, that would pay for a visit to another doctor. But these patients are willing to pay cash for the privilege of seeing a doctor who will spend extra time with them, will see them immediately, and can make a phone call to a specialist on their behalf if they have trouble getting past the primary care gatekeeper at their own health management organization. "I'm a facilitator, not just a doctor," Dawson says. He also is a safety valve for the already well-insured in our $1.7 trillion health care system. For his middle-class and upper-class patients, insurance alone isn't enough to assure peace of mind. They go outside the system to get help from Dawson.

Meanwhile, hundreds of thousands of low-income California families are ignoring the chance to buy a bargain, heavily subsidized health policy for their children through the state's Healthy Families program. It offers coverage at up to $9 a month per child, with a maximum of $27 a month regardless of the size of the family. "The policy has an actuarial value of $1,500, and yet they still won't sign up," says a health policy expert. (Let's call him Harry Samuels.) While many poor people don't realize their kids are eligible for government-subsidized health insurance and others are deterred by complicated enrollment forms, Samuels is frustrated that it's so hard to practically give away good coverage.

Dawson and Samuels are real, but they don't want their real names used, Dawson for reasons of privacy, and Samuels because he thinks that his colleagues in the foundation and academic worlds would ostracize him for casting doubt on the dream of universal health coverage through an insurance policy for all, rich and poor alike.

These two stories illustrate the complexity of moving the country toward a better health insurance system. On the one hand, if coverage is not comprehensive and immediate, it does not meet the type of care that many people want. On the other hand, many uninsured families, with competing demands on their limited resources, are unwilling or unable to pay insurance premiums even when low-cost coverage is available.

The Robert Wood Johnson Foundation works the same turf as Samuels, and has been pursuing the goal of universal access to health care since it opened for business in 1972. The biggest of all foundations dealing exclusively in the health field, Robert Wood Johnson disburses more than $400 million a year to improve health and health care in the United States. It is a vast sum for the nonprofit world, but relatively little in the grand scheme of things; the American health system spends nearly $5 billion *a day,* consuming about 15 percent of the entire output of goods and services in the national economy. Through leadership, inspiration, discussion, and a flow of grant money, the Robert Wood Johnson Foundation has been trying to bring about a nation in which everyone has access to good health care. Much of the time, this revolves around ideas for getting health insurance coverage for those who don't have it.

Stable, affordable health coverage for all Americans has been a consistent goal of the Foundation, and the inability to achieve it is the biggest failure, said Steven Schroeder, who was the Foundation's president from 1990 until 2002. This failure "was the single most bitter pill" of all Foundation efforts, he said. "It was the hardest by far. It broke our hearts."

Over 15 percent of the American population lacks health insurance, roughly the same percentage as when the Robert Wood Johnson Foundation began operating as a national philanthropy in 1972 and the same as in 1993, when President Clinton proposed a plan to provide health care for all. And the political climate today is more challenging and less receptive to the idea of government action to fashion a health care umbrella sheltering every American.

Although there is no universal care in America, the population is healthier than it has ever been. Between 1990 and 2003, there was a 34 percent drop in deaths from infectious disease, a 32 percent decline in infant mortality, and a 17 percent decline in deaths from heart disease.[1] Not only are people healthier but also the medical care system can do much more for them than it could just a generation ago. The first heart bypass operation was performed at the Cleveland Clinic in 1967, and now it is one of Medicare's routine procedures, even for people 85 and older. Cataract surgery once meant a week in the hospital, your head strapped to a rigid frame. Now it can be done as an outpatient procedure at an eye surgeon's office, and you can be playing tennis again in a couple of days.

The blessings of modern health care are unevenly distributed, however, and depend on the ability to pay for the care. The health care you get often comes down to the kind of job you have and the income of your family (the biggest single source of personal bankruptcies is medical expenses), and whether you have health insurance. The Foundation would like to see affordable health care for all Americans, giving them the security of knowing that they can pay the bills for a serious illness without going broke and that they can get the preventive care, such as routine checkups and immunizations, that will keep them healthy.

—ɯ— **Three Approaches**

The Foundation has taken a three-pronged approach to the issue of health insurance coverage, with the emphasis shifting at different times and represented by three different constituencies within the Foundation and the field of health policy.

First are ambitious reformers, who dream of changing the system so that everyone has health insurance coverage—something enjoyed by the citizens of every other industrial country. They have a big vision, pondering ways to get Congress and the president to place in the hands of the uninsured a card they can take to the doctor's office and the hospital with confidence that the bills will be paid.

The second group consists of hopeful pragmatists. They would like to solve the health care puzzle piece by discrete piece—a successful new primary care clinic here, an expanded school health program there, an enrollment drive for Medicaid in a third location. Washington may someday do the job, but people get sick right now and need help paying for their treatment, the hopeful pragmatists argue. Using this approach, the Foundation has funded a wide variety of programs since the 1980s, many of them designed to expand insurance coverage to children.

A third group is made up of numbers gurus, policy analysts who gather and examine information so that policymakers will know better how and where people get their health care services. The numbers gurus want to understand insurance markets, consumer behavior, and other arcane topics, and to offer the ambitious reformers and the hopeful pragmatists their analysis and numbers so they can work better and smarter.

Because of the work of the numbers gurus, we know a lot more about who the uninsured are, how they got that way, and how they move through and out of the system. We also have lots of information on the complexities of small group insurance, most of it discouraging. We know it is virtually impossible to design any plan to expand significantly the current level of coverage among small firms. "For many of them [the small businesses] any premium beyond zero dollars is too much," observed Jack Meyer, president of the Economic and Social Research Institute, in Washington, D.C., which has done considerable health policy research for the Foundation. The numbers gurus have produced lots of plans for covering the uninsured, courtesy of sophisticated thinkers underwritten by the Foundation. Many of those plans got an initial burst of publicity but are now gathering dust on the shelves in the offices of health care policy experts.

The Foundation has always featured a mixture of work from all three of these groups. Currently, the ambitious reformers seem to be forging ahead, powered by Cover the Uninsured Week, an unprecedented public education campaign to keep health care coverage on the national policy agenda. A recent draft statement by the Foundation's staff states: "Over three decades, the Foundation has commissioned a significant body of research and funded projects that have explored the potential of various local, state, and private sector options for expanding coverage. Results of its research and field work have led the Foundation to conclude that while health care is delivered locally, *it cannot be made available to all without a change in federal policy*" [italics added].

The ambitious reformers face a steep uphill climb. The current climate in Washington is daunting, with the president and Republican majorities in both houses of Congress seemingly averse to any far-reaching new federal health care coverage efforts. It will be even harder than in earlier years to figure out ways to spread the benefits of health care, because coverage is so much more costly than ever before, with a corporate policy for an individual exceeding $3,000 a year and a family policy costing about $10,000. "We must come to grips with the cost question," says Stuart Schear, a former senior communications officer at the Foundation, who oversaw the Foundation's campaign to make covering the uninsured a national political priority. "Health care is extraordinarily expensive, and in our next phase of work we will start research and analysis to look at what are the causes of the increase and what can be done to restrain them."

—ᴡᴡ— Reforming the System

The dream of bringing quality health care to everyone has been a recurring theme in American society, since long before the Robert Wood Johnson Foundation opened its doors in 1972. President Franklin Roosevelt had considered including health insurance in the package of proposals that eventually became the foundation of Social Security and unemployment insurance in 1935. But the idea was scrapped for fear of touching off a dispute with the American Medical Association, which regarded any government intrusion into the delivery of health care as socialized medicine. The idea surfaced again as a proposal from President Harry Truman. The AMA called it socialism and defeated it.

Medicare was created in 1965, bringing health insurance coverage to those over sixty-five and to disabled people of all ages. At the same time, Medicaid was created as a program enabling poor people to get health care. This burst of expansionary government funding of health care may have been a historical anomaly. The legacy of President John F. Kennedy, combined with the overwhelming electoral victory of Lyndon Johnson and the Democratic Party in 1964, created a spirit of enthusiastic activism that resulted in the passage of important social legislation.

For the vast majority of insured Americans, insurance through the workplace was and is the standard way to get health coverage. Your employer decides whether or not to offer health insurance and picks the plans from which you choose. The cost is tax-deductible for the company, and is not counted as income for the worker. The genesis of coverage at work was the World War II freeze on wages. To attract workers without increasing pay levels, Henry J. Kaiser, who was building ships for the Navy, offered free health coverage through a unique collection of Kaiser clinics, Kaiser owned-hospitals, and panels of doctors working full-time for Kaiser.

Health insurance coverage spread quickly after World War II; unions made health insurance a basic demand in their bargaining with the nation's large manufacturing companies. The benefit spread rapidly through industry, with both unionized and nonunion firms adopting it. Today, 61 percent of American workers are covered by employer-sponsored health insurance. The percentage ebbs and flows with the economy, but it is now declining, because the rapidly rising cost is putting health insurance beyond the reach of many small firms and many workers.

When the Robert Wood Johnson Foundation began its operations, during the Nixon Administration, policy experts believed, optimistically, that some form of national health insurance was just a few steps away from becoming a reality. "The uneven availability of continuing medical care of acceptable quality is one of the most serious problems we face today," David Rogers, the Foundation's first president, wrote in the 1972 *Annual Report.* "We need to better provide health services of the right kind, at the right time, to those who need it. Therefore, in its initial years, the foundation will try to identify and encourage efforts to expand and improve the delivery of primary, frontline care."

Confident that the system was heading toward national health coverage, the Foundation's early focus was on training the personnel who would be delivering the new health care services. It gave money to academic heath centers, funding new medical and dental students, residency programs in primary care and pediatrics, and training for nurse practitioners and physicians' assistants. A new cadre of Clinical Scholars and Health Policy Fellows was given financial support. The Foundation "supported programs that attracted talented young people at elite institutions and promulgated the importance of health services research, primary care, and public health," wrote two former Foundation executive vice presidents.[2]

Increasing access to care was the goal as the Foundation staff and grantees envisioned an expanded national system of care. But the vision of national health coverage as just around the corner dissipated by the middle of the decade. By 1980, it had become clear that cost was a formidable obstacle to attaining the goal of universal access.

During the 1980s, the Foundation's attention turned to the states—in part because many state governments wanted to expand health insurance (and reduce their own Medicaid costs) for their residents and partly because of the hope that models might be developed that could be used by other states or, eventually, by the federal government.

One approach the Foundation adopted was building coalitions of interested and influential organizations. Between 1981 and 1989, the Foundation funded the Community Programs for Affordable Health Care. Under this $14 million program, coalitions were formed among a broad range of interest groups, including business, labor, insurers, and hospital managers, to figure out ways to keep down the inflation of medical costs. Many experts believe that insurance coverage will expand only when health care costs are controlled. Eleven hospital sites received Foundation grants and technical assistance to help them figure out how they could save money while still providing first-rate care. But the program failed. Building coalitions turned out to be more difficult than originally envisioned, and the cost problem proved to be seemingly intractable, as it continues to be. "Effective cost containment strategies entail making tough choices, such as paying lower salaries, imposing restrictions, and contracting with certain doctors and not others," the medical journalist Carolyn Newbergh wrote. "But community leaders, who prefer to be known for expanding and improving their community's health care services, didn't want to gore anyone's ox."[3] Perhaps, though, the program did not succeed because it focused on the wrong level of government. As three Foundation officials wrote in 1990, "The program's central flaw, perhaps, was its misguided assumption that cost containment could be achieved through intervention at the community or local level, when the true levers of power and control existed (and still exist) at the national and state levels of the health care system."[4]

In 1985, the Foundation funded another state-oriented systems reform initiative, the Health Care for the Uninsured Program. It was designed to test innovative, incremental strategies for making health insurance coverage more available and affordable to small businesses. Under the $6.5 million program, fourteen states either developed new insurance products or subsidized existing ones. The Florida Health Access project, for example, used a state purchasing cooperative to lower premiums. The Arizona Health Care Group lowered premiums by subsidizing administrative and marketing costs. The state of Washington's Basic Health Plan used direct subsidies to provide coverage to low-income, uninsured individuals. There was a study of local insurance markets and underwriting practices. In addition, there was a major survey of more than 1,300 small companies with twenty-five or fewer workers at four sites—Denver; Flint, Michigan; Tampa; and Tucson.

The results from the program were revealing. The cost of insurance emerged as a major obstacle to small firms' purchasing health insurance for their employees. One lesson from the program was that health insurance, even if heavily subsidized, was unaffordable for small businesses. Writing in the journal *Health Affairs,* the program's evaluators observed, "Because of current underwriting practices, some small businesses would find it difficult to respond to any financial incentives or government mandates to provide health benefits to their employees."[5]

A second, and more disturbing, lesson to emerge from this program was that "there is a fairly hard-core group of small-business owners who do not want to provide health insurance benefits to their employees." This conclusion of the evaluators was buttressed by the statistic that "almost half the employers in our survey who do not offer health insurance indicated that they were not interested in doing so."[6] The relevance for national policy was highlighted in the conclusion of the program's directors that "efforts to expand the current employer-based insurance system are not likely to achieve universal financial access to health care without *requiring* [emphasis added] universal participation."[7]

These lessons seem to be resolutely ignored as policymakers proclaim the need for affordable new policies that will be bought by entrepreneurs eager to insure their employees. Foundation research has shown repeatedly that it is extremely hard to make progress with this approach. California, for example, established a special program to help the marketing of affordable policies to small businesses, with a wide range of choices on coverage and limits on prices. By the end of the 1990s, only 2 percent of the eligible firms in the state, with an aggregate workforce of 140,000 people, were participating. About 80 percent of them already had health insurance coverage, and their companies switched to the state-backed alliance to get better prices, according to Columbia University professors Lawrence Brown and Michael Sparer.[8]

The push for a national health care approach revived again in the 1990s. Harris Wofford, a Democrat running for a United States Senate seat in Pennsylvania, defeated the heavily favored Republican candidate, former U.S. attorney general Richard Thornburgh. Wofford surged in the polls after he made health care access his key issue, saying that if criminals are entitled to have a lawyer, voters should be guaranteed access to a doctor. With Wofford's victory, health care became a big issue in the next presidential campaign.

In 1992, Bill Clinton was elected president with a pledge to bring secure health care to all Americans. The Foundation was invited to help educate first lady Hillary Clinton and other key administration officials about the complexities of health care. Dozens of Foundation grantees were enlisted to testify at public sessions. The audience at various times included Mrs. Clinton, Tipper Gore, the wife of vice president Al Gore, and Donna Shalala, the secretary of Health and Human Services. There were sessions in Iowa, Michigan, and Florida, with the final one in Washington.

"Mrs. Clinton basically listened," Schroeder recalled. "It got tremendous media coverage and we were not prepared for it. We were kind of naïve. It was portrayed as a partisan issue. We said we were just helping people understand what was out there in the health field." The Foundation, and its staff and grantees, were accused of being a group of big-government liberals.

The accusation stung, and although Schroeder insists that the Foundation's trustees never told the staff to back away, the Foundation has been cautious in its approach since then. Although the Foundation's reticence is due, in large part, to its having been burned by its role during consideration of the Clinton health care reform plan, there are other factors too. The Foundation has a long-standing policy of emphasizing the visibility of its grantees rather than promulgating any plan that *it* favors. And the Foundation can't go too far in supporting any specific proposal without raising concern about losing credibility as a neutral source of unbiased information on health and health care.

With the failure of the Clinton health reform plan, the drive toward national reform dissipated. Employers asked for financial relief against rising health care costs, and insurance companies delivered with managed care mechanisms, moving millions of people into health maintenance organizations, or HMOs. Patients had to stay within designated networks of doctors and hospitals. Primary care doctors became gatekeepers for the system, and seeing a specialist without getting a referral sometimes became a lengthy bureaucratic process. The relentless inflation in health care costs was slowed, but there was a consumer backlash. Insurers were ordering hospitals to send women home within twenty-four hours after giving birth—a practice that was denounced in the press and ultimately banned by Congress. Employers and legislators were inundated with complaints, and they ordered the insurance plans to ease their restrictive practices. Managed care restraints were loosened, costs rose, and access again became an issue.

The Foundation had a creative response, prompted by Jack Ebeler, at the time a senior vice president of the Foundation. He talked with Ron Pollack, the executive director of Families USA, a liberal advocacy group, and Chip Kahn, then the president of the Health Insurance Association of America, an industry trade group. They had fought on opposite sides of the health policy wars for years but respected each other. The result was the convening of a "strange bedfellows conference" of disparate interest groups contending over the coverage issue. Everyone had a plan, a first choice to deal with the coverage crisis. The idea of convening the strange bedfellows was to get beyond the second choice—doing nothing—to find some common ground. The participating groups—including the U.S. Chamber of Commerce, the Service Employees International Union, the American Hospital Association, and the AFL-CIO—all could agree that the coverage issue was paramount and that everyone should have access to health care through insurance. Participants signed letters to Congress urging federal action to cover the uninsured. The strange bedfellows have continued to meet and to search for acceptable approaches to expanding coverage.

The Foundation decided to make a major commitment to bringing the issue beyond the Washington beltway to the broadest possible national audience. This led to Cover the Uninsured Week, in 2003, with hundreds of local events and campaigns to keep the spotlight on the plight of the millions of Americans who lacked coverage. The campaign heightened awareness. Polling by the Foundation showed that coverage had replaced costs as the top health issue, with 23 percent citing it compared with 16 percent a year before.[9]

In 2004, the Foundation funded a second Cover the Uninsured Week, which featured more than 2,700 local events, including all fifty states and the District of Columbia. More than 250 national organizations and 2,500 local groups were involved. There were rallies, health fairs, speeches, and theatrical depictions of the lives of the uninsured. The Foundation spent nearly $7 million and raised $2.6 million from other supporting organizations. A third Cover the Uninsured Week was held in May 2005.

The focus, however, was on the problem, rather than on specific solutions. Sometimes this was frustrating for participants in the awareness campaign, who wished to focus on specific remedies for the 800-pound-gorilla issue of cost.

Now, in 2006, comes the hard part for the Foundation and the nation—finding solutions to the problems trumpeted through Cover the Uninsured Week. "Action on the federal level is key to expanding coverage and making it affordable and stable for all Americans," a staff policy paper concluded. The circle has been closed, going back to 1972, when the Foundation began.

—᛭— Pragmatic and Incremental Approaches

Although the Foundation has looked to promote health care reform that could lead to universal coverage—and, in fact, it promises to judge its success by whether a national policy ensuring stable and affordable coverage for all has been adopted by 2010—the Foundation has simultaneously sought smaller-scale opportunities to expand insurance coverage. Most often, this incremental strategy focused on the states, which were seen as laboratories where new approaches to covering the uninsured could be developed and incubated. This was the essence of pragmatism—if we can't get the job done through national efforts, let's help the states get it done, one by one.

As one example, the findings from the earlier Health Care for the Uninsured program indicated that small businesses would not provide coverage for their employees, even if offered price breaks (a concept at the heart of a number of federal health reform proposals). As a follow-up, the Foundation funded a variation of the program called State Coverage Initiatives. Under the new program, which was authorized in 1992, state governments received grants to test ways that they can increase health insurance coverage. For example:

- Arkansas created a buy-in for small employers to get coverage for their low-paid workers under the state's Medicaid program.

- New Mexico devised a basic benefits package for small companies, with the state acting as a vendor and collector of premiums to keep down administrative costs.

- Oregon received help with a federal waiver to expand its Medicaid program to cover more people.

- Rhode Island had a program to provide insurance for low-income families.

In the mid-1990s, with the failure of the Clinton health reform plan having dealt a severe blow to the possibility of universal health care, the Foundation was searching for new ways to expand health insurance coverage. One way was to provide coverage for children, a group that the Foundation had been concerned with for many years. In 1990, the Foundation had funded a Healthy Kids program in Florida, which used subsidized insurance, initially through schools, to bring coverage to more than 60,000 children. With additional funds from the Foundation, the Florida approach, with variations, was replicated in a number of states.[10]

Building on its experience in funding innovative ways to bring health insurance to children, the Foundation in 1997 developed a new $13 million three-year initiative called Covering Kids that would help local coalitions in fifteen states try to identify children eligible for Medicaid and sign them up. Covering Kids came just as Congress was considering a new health insurance program for children, the State Children's Health Insurance Program, or SCHIP, which was eventually passed as part of the Balanced Budget Act of 1997. Senator Edward M. Kennedy, a liberal Democrat, and Senator Orrin Hatch, a conservative Republican, sent their staff members out of a meeting on Capitol Hill, shut the door, and worked out a deal to provide generous funding to the states to provide health insurance for children. States had the choice of expanding eligibility under the current Medicaid program, creating a new health program for children, or doing some of each.

Suddenly there was new government support and resources for expanded health access, and the Foundation seized the opportunity to support the federal effort to expand coverage for children. In 1998, the Foundation authorized an additional $34 million to transform the Covering Kids program into a nationwide effort, with projects in every state and the District of Columbia. One hundred seventy-three pilot projects, and 4,200 public and private organizations, joined coalitions to enroll eligible but unregistered children in Medicaid and SCHIP by developing simplified application forms, doing outreach, and persuading state officials to reduce restrictions such as means tests and in-person interviews.

As private insurance coverage has diminished in the past three years, Medicaid and SCHIP have filled the gap, at least for children. The proportion of the population covered by employer-sponsored insurance fell from 67 percent to 63 percent between 2001 and 2003, but the proportion of low-income children covered by the public programs rose sharply—from 38 percent to 49 percent—an increase of almost five million children. According to a report by the Center for Studying Health System Change, a research group funded by the Foundation, "Public insurance clearly picked up the slack as the United States moved through a recession and jobless recovery and employer coverage declined. SCHIP, enacted in 1997, played a major role and has been remarkably successful in providing a safety net to children who otherwise might be uninsured."[11]

Steven Schroeder considers the Foundation's role in increasing the enrollment of children as one the Foundation's greatest accomplishments. Much of the expansion in kids' coverage is due to the billions invested by the federal and state governments. But as the program's evaluators noted,

> Unquestionably there are children with health coverage now who would not
> have had coverage except for the efforts of state and local Covering Kids initiative

grantees. It is not possible, of course, to isolate the exact number. It is worth noting, however, that during the period that the Covering Kids initiative has been operational, a downward trend in the number of children enrolled in Medicaid reversed and began to increase. Furthermore, enrollment in SCHIP has increased dramatically since the first program was implemented in 1998. Federal reports indicate that more than three million children were covered by SCHIP during fiscal year 2000.[12]

In addition, the evaluators reported, "Covering Kids had served as a change agent in many states, and had encouraged a fundamental change in states' perception of the Medicaid program—from a welfare program to a health insurance program with a consumer focus. Furthermore, the program had generated groups of individuals in each state who were now knowledgeable about Medicaid eligibility to an extent that would not have been possible without the Covering Kids initiative."

Some states have expanded eligibility to the parents of children enrolled in SCHIP. In 2001, to take advantage of federal revenues available for this new family eligibility, the Foundation expanded Covering Kids into Covering Kids & Families, a five-year $65 million program. The Southern Institute on Children and Families, which administers the programs, has worked closely with state officials in fashioning programs that will allow the parents of SCHIP children to be covered by governmental health insurance.

Yet these programs threaten to become victims of their own success. Medicaid costs are growing far faster than the tax revenues of the states, which pay anywhere from 17 percent to 50 percent of total program costs. Medicaid, which consumed about 8 percent of state budgets a generation ago, is now verging on 25 percent—an intolerably large figure for many states. As the Medicaid and SCHIP programs enroll more children and their parents, the costs to the states rise and the strain on precious state resources increases. Even though spending for children's health care consumes a relatively modest share of state Medicaid budgets (most children are healthy most of the time), some states have tried to curb the growth in spending by making it harder for parents to enroll their children. Among the tools some states have used are a temporary freeze on new enrollment and a requirement to be re-certified for eligibility every six months instead of yearly.

—ɯ— Collecting and Analyzing Data

Meanwhile, the Foundation has been supporting organizations and individuals who have been steadily and often quietly producing a variety of reports that help policymakers and the public understand some of the complexities of the health care system, and that suggest just how hard it will be for the Foundation to achieve its long-sought goal of access to health care for every American. Organizations include

- Changes in Health Care Financing and Organization, or HCFO. Headquartered at AcademyHealth in Washington, D.C., HCFO has been funded since 1988. It awards grants to researchers whose research is aimed at providing reliable information for policymakers and public officials as they reshape the health care system. HCFO replaced the Program for Demonstration and Research on Health Care Costs, which the Foundation had funded between 1982 and 1987, but which evaluators considered to be too limited because of its focus on clinical data.

- The Center for Studying Health System Change. The Center provides insights both at the macro level, looking at the whole structure of the intricate national web of health care, and the micro level, periodic visits and in-depth reports about the widely divergent health care markets in twelve communities. Along with its other research, the Center tracks changes over time. It conducted a baseline study in 1996–1997, encompassing 32,000 households, 12,000 doctors, and 22,000 employers at sixty random sites. The study is repeated periodically, providing a wealth of information on health coverage, costs, and trends.[13]

- The State Health Access Data Assistance Center, or SHADAC, at the University of Minnesota. SHADAC supports the development of state-specific data sets and analysis on issues of health insurance coverage.

- The Economic Research Initiative on the Uninsured at the University of Michigan. This organization carries out and publishes economic research on health insurance. It has done extensive research on the dynamics of insurance coverage and the effect of being uninsured.

- The Urban Institute's National Survey of America's Families. The Urban Institute surveyed families in thirteen states, providing a comprehensive look at the well-being of children and adults under sixty-five. It studies issues of access and health insurance coverage among low-income families.

- The Economic and Social Research Institute, in Washington, D.C. The Institute conducts a wide range of research on health and social policy. Its recent publications include reports on safety net hospitals, strategies for covering the uninsured, and Medicaid coverage for poor adults.

- The Institute of Medicine. The IOM has produced six reports on the consequences of being uninsured.

The Foundation has gone beyond the gathering of facts illuminating the health care system and has ventured into the area of "what if," looking at the statistical basis of a universal health care system and how it might be structured. According to a Foundation-commissioned report by the Economic and Social Research Institute, covering all the uninsured would cost between $75 billion and $150 billion a year. The report, entitled *Covering America: Real Remedies for the Uninsured,* showed a broad and imaginative range of thinking from liberal to centrist to conservative. One author proposed a combination of an individual mandate and tax credits whereby all Americans would have to maintain a basic level of coverage. Tax credits would assure that they spent no more than 10 percent of income for their insurance coverage. Another suggested repealing the tax-free status of health insurance premiums paid by employers and employees, with the resulting billions of dollars in tax revenues going to the states to help low-income families buy health insurance. Another called for the expansion of Medicaid and the State Children's Health Insurance Program, combined with tax credits, to encourage small firms to offer coverage.

These reports, and others like them, represent serious thinking. Yet there is a danger that they will remain unread except by aficionados of the health care debate and thus be limited in their influence. In recent years, the Foundation has expanded its efforts to communicate findings from its grantees' research through vehicles such as an expanded Web site, support for grantee Web sites, convening of meetings of leading thinkers and actors in health insurance, and support of the journal *Health Affairs*. The Foundation also has funded an initiative to analyze the research on specific health policy issues and summarize the conclusions that it is possible to draw based on the research. Syntheses of existing research have been done on topics such as ways to make individual health insurance policies more affordable, how to reduce health insurance premiums for small businesses, and whether increasing publicly funded health insurance would reduce the need for private insurance.

Despite these efforts, such reports appear to have had limited influence on the debate. This seems to be a persistent theme in the Foundation's work toward the goal of universal coverage. It assembles ideas and information and then fails to promote them aggressively. Although it has endorsed a set of general principles enunciated by the Institute of Medicine for "guiding the debate,"[14] the Foundation has been reluctant to support aggressively any particular approach that might lead to stable and affordable coverage for all Americans.

—w— Conclusion

The Foundation's approach to covering the uninsured has shifted as the national discussion has ebbed and flowed from worries about access to fears about runaway costs. Its most noteworthy achievements so far in bringing about expanded coverage have been at the margin—promoting and publicizing the availability of government health insurance for children and their parents, helping state and local officials do a better job of administering the programs under their control, stimulating state experiments in coverage, prodding them to take advantage whenever there are more federal dollars to disburse, giving training and enthusiasm to the local activists who labor on these issues, and keeping the issue of health insurance alive through public communications campaigns.

At the same time, the Foundation has supported the generation of a vast amount of data to help deepen understanding of how the health care system works and to examine ideas for expanding health insurance coverage. What is not certain is whether this knowledge and these ideas help shape the debate. They are disseminated to and known by experts, but will policymakers and government officials choose to use them? The Foundation itself seems reluctant to inject itself more actively into the policy debate by promoting solutions, perhaps out of concern that it might be accused of stepping over the line and lobbying or perhaps for fear of risking its reputational capital.

Many of the Foundation's staff members and many of its grantees have had visions of the magical day when every American would have a card guaranteeing admittance to the doctor's office or the hospital without fear of going bankrupt. But these dreams have gone unrealized. There has not been a broad, consistent constituency among the nation's policymakers for such expansive notions of health reform. The Foundation has been constrained in efforts to push in that direction. It is, after all, a vehicle of philanthropy dependent on the tax code, not a political animal or an activist caucus. Yet the Foundation now has a strategic objective of stable and affordable health care coverage for all Americans by 2010. This has been the impossible dream so far. Can it become a reality now?

Notes

1. *America's Health: State Health Rankings.* United Health Foundation, American Public Health Association, and Partnership for Prevention, 2003, p. 14.
2. Sandy, L. G., and Reynolds, R. "Influencing Academic Health Centers, The Robert Wood Johnson Foundation Experience." *To Improve Health and Health Care 1998–1999: The Robert Wood Johnson Foundation Anthology.* San Francisco: Jossey-Bass, 1998.
3. Newbergh, C. "The Robert Wood Johnson Foundation's Efforts to Contain Health Care Costs." *To Improve Health and Health Care, Vol. VII: The Robert Wood Johnson Foundation Anthology.* San Francisco: Jossey-Bass, 2004.
4. Schroeder, S. A., Cohen, A., and Cantor, J. "Perspectives: The Funders." *Health Affairs,* 1990, *9,* pp. 29–33.
5. Zellers, W. K., McLaughlin, C. G., and Frick, K. D. "Small-Business Health Insurance: Only the Healthy Need Apply." *Health Affairs,* 1992, *11,* pp. 174–180.
6. McLaughlin, C. G., and Zellers, W. K. "The Shortcomings of Voluntarism in the Small-Group Insurance Market." *Health Affairs,* 1992, *11,* pp. 28–40.

7. Helms, W. D., Gauthier, A. K., and Campion, D. M. "Mending the Flaws in the Small-Group Market." *Health Affairs,* 1992, *11,* pp. 7–27.

8. Brown, L. D., and Sparer, M. "Window Shopping: State Health Reform Politics in the 1990s." *Health Affairs,* 2001, *20*(1), p. 55.

9. Brown, M. Robert Wood Johnson Foundation Report on Cover the Uninsured Week, forthcoming, p. 33.

10. Holloway, M. "Expanding Health Insurance for Children." *To Improve Health and Health Care 2000: The Robert Wood Johnson Foundation Anthology.* San Francisco: Jossey-Bass, 1999.

11. Strunk, B. C., and Reschovsky, J. D. "Trends in U.S. Heath Insurance Coverage, 2001–2003." *Tracking Report, Insurance Coverage and Costs, Results from the Community Tracking Study, 2004, 9.* Washington, D.C.: Center for Studying Health System Change.

12. Health Management Associates. *Covering Kids Initiative Assessment Project, Final Report,* January 19, 2001, p. 4.

13. Newbergh, C. "The Health Tracking Initiative." *To Improve Health and Health Care, Vol. VI: The Robert Wood Johnson Foundation Anthology.* San Francisco: Jossey-Bass, 2003.

14. Institute of Medicine. *Insuring America's Health: Principles and Recommendations.* Washington, D.C.: National Academies Press, 2004.

Appendix. Initiatives to Cover the Uninsured

Center for Studying Health System Change (Health Tracking): $134,000,000

Changes in Health Care Financing and Organization: $76,400,000

Covering Kids & Families: $65,000,000

Covering Kids: $47,000,000

State Coverage Initiatives: $42,900,000

Communities in Charge: $16,800,000

Assessing the New Federalism: $16,600,000

Urban Institute National Study of American Families: $16,000,000

Cover the Uninsured Week: $11,400,000

Research Initiative on Health Insurance: $9,800,000

Covering America (Grants to Economic and Social Research Institute): $7,000,000

Support for Project Hope and the Health Affairs Journal: $5,000,000

SHADAC: $5,000,000

IOM Reports: $3,700,000

Annual Health Coverage Conferences, D.C.: $2,400,000

Healthy Kids Replication: $1,200,000

Community Programs for Affordable Health Care: $14,000,000

Health Care for the Uninsured: $6,500,000

Healthy Kids Pilot: $200,000

Amount (in millions)

$130
$70
$60
$50
$40
$30
$20
$10
$0

1980   1985   1990   1995   2000   2005

Year

The Robert Wood Johnson Foundation's Safety Net Programs

James Bornemeier

Editors' Introduction

The term *safety net,* which entered the health care vernacular during the Reagan administration, means different things to different people. To some, it is code for an alternative—and unsatisfactory—approach to caring for the poor: a parallel system of health services in lieu of a universal health insurance system. To others, it refers to providers of health care for people who live in low-income urban or remote rural locations where mainstream providers often do not locate. In the latter sense, an effective safety net will still be needed even when low-income, vulnerable populations have insurance coverage.

This chapter flows naturally from the previous chapter on the Robert Wood Johnson Foundation's efforts to expand health insurance coverage. For even as the Foundation has worked to expand such coverage, it has also funded initiatives to bring services to needy people—safety net services.

Successful safety net programs can undermine the case for universal health insurance. Because of this, plus the difficulty reaching agreement on exactly what the safety net consists of and the strong partisan feelings the term engenders, it is not surprising that the chapter's author, James Bornemeier, a freelance writer specializing in health and social policy issues, finds that the Foundation's approach to the safety net, though serious, has been inconsistent. Nonetheless, in examining Foundation-funded programs to maintain the safety net, Bornemeier highlights a number of interesting and worthwhile initiatives that have provided services to people who otherwise would not have received them. And even though the Foundation has never specified maintaining the safety net as a priority, it is striving, within its current impact framework, to improve the care given to vulnerable populations and to reduce the disparity in the quality of health care received by racial and ethnic minorities.

—m— **I**n the United States, the term *safety net* has come to mean the patchwork of health care providers and social service agencies—public hospitals, community health centers, local clinics, and some primary care physicians—that offers a combination of medical care and other services, such as language translation and transportation, to uninsured and vulnerable citizens. A recent report of the Institute of Medicine observed, "The safety net is the default system of care for many of the forty-four million low-income Americans with no or limited health insurance, as well as many Medicaid beneficiaries and people with special needs."[1] In the absence of universal insurance coverage, it seems likely that the nation will continue to rely on safety net providers to care for its most disadvantaged populations. For the Robert Wood Johnson Foundation, this fact of life has provided the backdrop for a number of programs that have sought to strengthen this often overwhelmed segment of the health care system.

Yet the Foundation's diverse safety net efforts, for all their ingenuity and earnestness, have never been consistently coordinated under a grand strategy (and certainly never anointed with an eponymous portfolio), and over the Foundation's existence, engagement with safety net issues has taken place episodically and some would say erratically.

To understand why, it's instructive to return to the Foundation's earliest years and recall a political consensus that by today's starkly divided electorate seems nearly unimaginable. In 1972, legislation to establish national health insurance was wending its way through Congress. Massachusetts Senator Edward Kennedy, chairman of the Health Subcommittee, was pushing the bill forward in the Senate, while Representative Wilbur Mills of Arkansas, chairman of the Ways and Means Committee, was shepherding it through the House. President Richard Nixon supported the concept. Though passage of the legislation was by no means certain, some form of national health insurance seemed likely.

"The notion of extending health insurance to the entire population didn't seem as farfetched as it does now," recalls Paul Jellinek, a former Foundation vice president. "The Foundation believed that health insurance was right around the corner, and the real challenge was to have a supply of doctors who could actually deliver the care. What good would it do for everyone to have an insurance card if there were no doctors to take it to?"

Access to care was a growing issue, and the Foundation's board, anticipating the historic adoption of universal coverage, was poised to assist in the flowering of this new health care paradigm. "They wanted to get behind something that the average American would understand and approve of," Jellinek says.

The legislative moment was lost. Mills began flaunting his enthusiasm for an Argentine ecdysiast, and his career derailed. Nixon had become embroiled in the Watergate scandal, leaving him little time to worry about health care. By the time of Nixon's resignation, in 1974, the momentum for national health insurance had passed.

Larger forces were also at work. A more conservative strain of Republican national leader, exemplified by California's Governor Ronald Reagan, was on the rise—one who took a sharply different view of the role of the federal government. Robert Blendon, a Foundation vice president from 1971 to 1986, recalls, "Reagan thought that Nixon was nuts and that Republicans should not be for these large government systems. He thought we should turn it over to the states and get the federal government out of trying to fix these problems."

"We were quite affected by the shift in the national mood," says Blendon, now a professor at the Harvard School of Public Health and the John F. Kennedy School of Government. "The country was faced with a lot of problems but Reagan believed it wasn't the federal government's responsibility to solve them. We at the Foundation thought we were going to be involved in numerous programs and partnerships, but quite quickly all these possibilities left the scene."

"The Foundation found itself all dressed up with no place to go," Jellinek says, "and it was confused about what it should do."

"Access to care was the focus," Blendon says. "We wanted to put together systems that tried to improve access for people who were having really difficult problems." But the term *safety net* was not invoked.

As the prospect of national health insurance faded from view and the role of government diminished, the Foundation had to readjust its relationship with the safety net. "They struggled for seven or eight years to fig-ure out what they wanted to do," says John Billings, a Foundation grantee and director of the Center for Health and Public Service Research at New York University and professor of health policy at the Robert F. Wagner Graduate School of Public Service. "They couldn't decide if the safety net providers were part of the problem or part of the answer. A lot of people thought that the safety net providers hadn't been performing very well and that they had to be really shaken up. Therefore, doing any program directed at the current players didn't make much sense. That sort of par-alyzed them for a while." The result? "They never developed a very clear, explicit, or coherent approach to what they wanted to do about improv-ing the performance of the safety net," Billings says.

Along with concerns about the performance of safety net providers, the Foundation's approach to the safety net was complicated by a conun-drum: Improving the quality and the delivery of safety net care gives com-fort to those who argue against universal coverage. "We have a goal of increasing access to care, and we believe across the Foundation that the single strongest, most powerful tool toward access is health insurance," says Pamela Dickson, a Foundation senior program officer. "We also rec-ognize that in the short term it's an impractical notion to assume that we are going to be able to get everybody covered by health insurance."

"From a practical point of view, we want to be helpful to efforts that provide services to people who are not going to have health insurance or aren't eligible for it," Dickson continued. "But when you support safety net efforts, you can become vulnerable to the argument that you don't need universal health insurance because the safety net is an adequate substitute. As a whole, the Foundation does not want to support that. That is one rea-son that the efforts to support safety nets may seem kind of sporadic."

Dickson's colleague, Anne Weiss, also a senior program officer at the Robert Wood Johnson Foundation, echoes these thoughts:

> When we first started thinking about safety net projects, we thought of them
> as related to the goal of access to health care: A lot of people get access to health
> care through the safety net, so let's see how we can make it supply more and
> better access. At some point in the late 1990s, our board and our leadership

coalesced around the idea of coverage—covering the uninsured. That positioned these safety net programs somewhat separately. We didn't want to suggest they were the solutions. To a certain extent, we wanted to suggest to people that these safety net programs demonstrated the inadequacy of local solutions and the need for a national solution. The Foundation shifted from being proactive, "Here's something we're doing and we hope more people will do it," to "Here's something we're doing to take a very tough look at the limitations of these strategies." That made safety net programs kind of an orphan for a while.

Despite the notion that successful safety net programs can potentially undermine the justification for universal health insurance, from the 1970s through much of the 1990s, the Foundation put forth an impressive array of initiatives that attacked nagging problems of inadequate, poor-quality, or inefficient health care for the nation's most vulnerable individuals. During those years, the Foundation developed national programs aimed at strengthening health care centers, improving access to care for the rural poor, assisting large cities in providing municipal health services, helping low-income people get proper dental care, and providing housing and health care to the homeless.

In 1999, the Foundation reorganized into teams, and safety net programs fell loosely under the auspices of the Priority Populations team, whose mission was to reduce nonfinancial barriers to health care. "We didn't call ourselves the safety net team," Dickson says, "but in a way we were looking at the barriers that, in addition to lack of coverage, block poor people from getting the health care they needed. 'Safety net' was there under the surface, but we didn't use it directly to describe our work."

In January 2003, Risa Lavizzo-Mourey became the president and chief executive officer of the Robert Wood Johnson Foundation. She quickly reorganized the Foundation into issue portfolios by employing an "impact framework" to heighten the emphasis on goals and results. Lavizzo-Mourey says:

The safety net plays out in several different ways in the impact framework. First, in the Vulnerable Populations portfolio, which is focused on providing innovative programs for the most vulnerable in our society. That's the same population that the safety net institutions typically serve. Second, in our Disparities team, which has as an objective to define evidence-based ways to reduce the disparities in health care based on race and ethnicity. Many of the ways in which the safety net institutions have been leaders is in providing care that addresses the disparities that people have both before and after they get health insurance. Last, and more significant for the overall economic viability of the safety net, we're continuing to push very hard to ensure that everyone has health insurance. Those three approaches to the kinds of populations and challenges that the safety net institutions address are the ways that we are demonstrating our strong commitment.

Lavizzo-Mourey notes that the new arrangement offers a more comprehensive strategy. "Before, there was a group of individuals [the Priority Populations team]that focused on some safety net issues, and there were very strong programs geared toward individual issues within the safety net, but there wasn't any multipronged approach that looked at the various challenges that safety net institutions have—financing, delivering high-quality care to an ethnically diverse population, and being located near and serving the most vulnerable people. The difference now is that we are looking at issues of the safety net from a multipronged approach."

—⟋⟋⟍—Notable Safety Net Programs

Writ large, the Foundation's safety net grantmaking has been aimed at expanding health care services for people who are poor or uninsured or who have difficulty gaining access to the system—minorities, people with serious mental illnesses, immigrants, and individuals living in inner cities or rural areas or having a disease such as AIDS. In this macro sense, virtually all the Foundation's programs could qualify as safety net programs.

But a tighter focus can be used: those programs aimed at providing or expanding medical services to individuals having difficulty getting adequate care because they are poor or uninsured or live in areas where physicians are in short supply. Even using this tighter focus, there is a rich lode of grantmaking initiatives. Here, grouped under the general categories of expanding ambulatory care, strengthening volunteerism, and improving services for homeless people, are sketches of some notable initiatives.

Expanding Ambulatory Care

Municipal Health Services Program (1977–1984, $15 million)

The Municipal Health Services Program was designed to respond to the increasing need for general medical care in urban communities, where municipal health departments and hospitals are the principal institutional resources available. The country's fifty largest cities were invited to apply for funding, and five—Baltimore, Cincinnati, Milwaukee, San Jose, and St. Louis—were selected to participate. The goal was to assist the cities in their efforts to provide basic health care services to families living in underserved urban neighborhoods. A key feature of the program was helping municipalities develop those services by consolidating and building upon existing services offered by public health departments, hospitals, and other local health agencies, with a limited investment in new funds by the municipality. It was developed in cooperation with the American Medical Association and the U.S. Conference of Mayors.[2]

One of the central questions Municipal Health Services sought to answer was this: Can the program improve access to care while containing costs to the Medicaid program? (The federal Health Care Financing Administration authorized waivers so that people could use primary care centers rather than more expensive hospital-based sources of care.) According to evaluators, the program had mixed success. In terms of access, the Municipal Health Services Program was able to provide certain targeted groups with sources of care, which were generally more convenient than those they had been using. But the program did not provide care at a lower cost than that received by people who went to other public facilities. "Costs overall were not significantly different for the Municipal Health Services Program and public facility users," the evaluators concluded, "[but] we are relatively certain that MHSP did not cost *more*."[3]

Program to Strengthen Primary Care Health Centers (1985–1994, $3.4 million)

In the early 1980s, a trend toward the privatization of health care led to a reduction in funding available to community health centers (which were called "primary care health centers" under the program), which had originated in the antipoverty programs of the 1960s as places where financially, medically, and geographically disadvantaged people could go for care. In response to this retrenchment, the Foundation developed the Program to Strengthen Primary Care Health Centers—specifically to help them become more entrepreneurial and less dependent on public funds. The program aimed at helping health centers find new sources of revenue and become more financially efficient. More precisely, it provided grants and technical assistance aimed at improving the operational, financial planning, and managerial capacities of health centers and reducing their dependence on federal support.

The activities initiated by the health centers focused on five major objectives:

- Increasing patient service revenues
- Serving more patients
- Promoting the stability of center operations
- Expanding the kinds of services provided at the centers
- Enhancing nonpatient revenues

According to the program's evaluation, those centers receiving Foundation support improved their financial stability. Most striking, one comparison center went bankrupt during the study period, but none of the participating centers met that fate.[4]

Hospital-based Rural Health Care Program
(1986–1992, $16.5 million)

A significant number of the 2,700 rural hospitals in the United States experience financial distress. Although closing may be appropriate for some, a large number are a vital part of their local communities. Rural hospitals are often a major capital investment, a large local employer, and an important provider of care for the poor and the elderly, and are necessary to recruiting and retaining physicians.[5]

The underlying assumption of the Foundation in this demonstration project was that local hospitals and their managers are a key leadership force in improving rural health care, and that small rural hospitals can accomplish more by working together with other hospitals than they can in isolation. In 1988, the Foundation initiated the Hospital-based Rural Health Care Program to improve the access, quality, and cost-efficiency of health services for rural populations by supporting consortia of hospitals to implement several strategies:

- Improve organizational arrangements by forming linkages among hospitals and other providers

- Promote cost-efficiency through improved management by sharing data and billing systems, management teams, the purchase of supplies and new technology, and the recruitment and employment of physicians and specialized staff

- Expand new revenue bases by diversifying into new health and health-related services, developing joint ventures, and expanding the use of existing systems

The response to the announcement of the program was overwhelming—some 180 applications were received. The program provided grants for up to four years, averaging about $625,000 a year to thirteen consortia of hospitals in rural areas. Examples of innovative consortia programs included efforts to provide a network of geriatric care providers in the western part of North Carolina; a hospital conversion from medical-surgical to psychiatric inpatient services in northeastern New York; and the cooperative recruitment of physicians by twelve hospitals in western New York and twenty hospitals in Wisconsin.

An evaluation by the University of Minnesota's Institute for Health Services Research found that nearly 40 percent of the networks had ceased to function within one year after the grant funding of the Robert Wood Johnson Foundation had ended, in 1991. The evaluators found that lack of funds was the precipitating factor in the demise of two-thirds of the networks. One out of five networks singled out competitive factors in explaining why they disbanded, for example, their fear of sharing information or resources with hospitals viewed as competitors for patients or outside funding. This suggested to the evaluators that "the rural hospital network is a relatively unstable organizational form."

Communities in Charge (1997–2005, $15.5 million)

In 1996, the Robert Wood Johnson Foundation provided partial support to the federal Health Resources and Services Administration for a national competition to identify and showcase innovative projects for delivering primary health care to underserved and vulnerable populations in local communities. One of the winners of that competition was the Hillsborough County Health Care Plan, a community-wide effort in Hillsborough County, Florida (which includes Tampa and surrounding communities), that resulted in a program that raised the local sales tax to finance a managed-care plan for 30,000 uninsured people. The Hillsborough model, which won an Innovations in Government award in 1995, was particularly interesting not only for its tax mechanism but also because it was a rare county-based approach whose scale seemed transferable elsewhere.

The Hillsborough County Health Care Plan inspired the Robert Wood Johnson Foundation to develop a new initiative that would encourage other communities to develop innovative programs for improving access and quality of care for their uninsured residents. Called Communities in Charge, the initiative was a competitive grants program that challenged local communities to rethink how funds and services are organized for the uninsured. It also provided funding and technical assistance to help communities design and implement new, or significantly expand existing, community-based approaches to the problem.[6]

Twenty communities received organizational and planning grants beginning in January 2000. Grants for development and implementation matching grants were awarded in January 2001 to fourteen communities. During the course of the program, the focus of Communities in Charge shifted, in part because of the economic downturn, surging state budget deficits, and increases in the number of uninsured, and in part because of the recognition that Hillsborough County's coverage program was an anomaly—an almost perfect meshing of state, county, and community political will—and that communities cannot solve the coverage problem without significant assistance from state and federal governments. The program was able to recommend smaller-bore strategies that had a better chance of being replicated (health policy forums, shared clinical records, state-federal partnership coverage programs) and strategies to be avoided (such as models requiring small businesses to buy insurance for their employees).

Pipeline, Profession, and Practice: Community-based Dental Education (2001–2007, $19 million)

Oral Health in America: A Report of the Surgeon General, released in May 2000, recognized impressive gains in oral health over the past fifty years for many Americans, but noted that only 35 percent of the people below the poverty line had visited a dentist in the previous year. It also noted that, sadly but not surprisingly, vulnerable populations—the poor, the medically disabled, the geographically isolated—suffered the worst oral health.[7]

The report cited several factors contributing to this disparity: public and voluntary dental clinics for low-income patients treat only seven million people a year of the tens of millions who are without adequate access to other care; the dental profession lacks the cultural and ethnic diversity necessary to enhance access to and utilization of oral health care by racial and ethnic minorities; and high tuition and the prospect of high student debt contribute to the decline in dental students from lower-income families.

The Pipeline, Profession, and Practice: Community-Based Dental Education program strives to increase access to dental care for underserved populations in urban and rural communities by expanding the number of underrepresented minority and low-income students studying dentistry. Specifically, the program is funding fifteen dental schools to, among other things, initiate programs to recruit, enroll, and graduate greater numbers of underrepresented minority and low-income students; change the standard curriculum to incorporate more public health dentistry training; raise awareness of sociocultural issues and sensitivity in the practice of dentistry; and advocate public policy changes at the national, state, and local levels. (The program is cofunded by the California Endowment, which supports participating dental schools in California.)

As an example, as part of the program at the University of North Carolina, dental students can do their required community training at sites that include prisons, nursing homes, psychiatric hospitals, veterans hospitals, mental institutions, and community health centers. As another example, the Temple School of Dentistry appointed an associate dean for institutional relations and community affairs to further develop and implement community-based programs. These programs now serve hundreds of underserved patients in Philadelphia and Tioga County, Pennsylvania. Community clinical rotations have become a requirement for graduation.

State Action for Oral Health Access (2001–2005, $8.2 million)

This program supports demonstration projects testing innovative approaches to expanding access to dental care for low-income, minority, and disabled individuals served through Medicaid, the State Children's Health Insurance Program, and the public health system. In South Carolina, for example, the Department of Health and Environmental Control developed a collaboration with a district African Methodist Episcopal Church in which children attending church events are screened and, where appropriate, referred to dentists. In Oregon, the Department of Human Services and the Oregon Dental Association developed a project whereby a coalition of public, volunteer, and professionals are working together to coordinate free or low-cost oral health services for low-income families.

Urgent Matters (2002–2007, $6.4 million)

Dramatic increases in emergency room wait times plague many big cities, with implications for the health and health care of millions. In a 2002 national survey, 62 percent of all American hospitals reported being at or over operating capacity in their emergency departments, and the number rose to 79 percent for urban hospitals.[8]

This situation is troubling, given the unique role of emergency departments in the health care system. Emergency rooms are often the only open door in a community's health care system and the only provider of many essential services, such as burn and trauma care. In addition, the nation's ability to respond to bioterrorism or events involving mass catastrophes requires both robust and sustainable hospital and emergency room capacity.

To help address these nagging problems, the Foundation funded Urgent Matters, an initiative to help hospitals relieve emergency room crowding. The program provides resources to hospitals in ten communities to improve the timeliness and the availability of emergency care. The hospitals work as part of a learning network to develop and implement best practices to maximize patient flow and relieve emergency room crowding. Four of the hospitals also received $250,000 for special demonstration projects to lessen emergency room crowding. All sites participate in a safety net assessment and community education process in conjunction with community partners. This helps raise awareness about the state of the local safety net.

Urgent Matters communicates program findings and lessons learned to a variety of local and national audiences. Beginning in February 2005, Urgent Matters embarked on its second phase, using seminars conducted over the Web, conferences, and a new learning network.

Strengthening Volunteerism

Reach Out (1993–1999, $11 million)

Against the backdrop of the failed health care reform efforts during the first Clinton administration, the Foundation unveiled a program designed to encourage locally based groups of physicians to volunteer their time to serve people without health insurance. Its official name: Reach Out: Physicians' Initiative to Expand Care to Underserved Americans.[9] Thirty-nine sites, ranging from entire states to inner cities to remote rural areas, received funds to increase access to care through a combination of physician leadership and community support. The two most common models—the free clinic and the referral network—accounted for two-thirds of the total number of projects.

As cited in the *Journal of the American Medical Society* in January 2000, approximately 11,000 physicians participated in Reach Out. Some 200,000 people received medical care through the program. Put differently, under Reach Out, approximately 2 percent of American physicians volunteered to treat 0.5 percent of the nation's uninsured. A significant number of these patients were provided with ongoing medical homes throughout the three-year implementation phase of the program, while others received specialized care such as surgery or costly tests.

In the view of H. Denman Scott, the program's director, Reach Out's most important accomplishment was probably its documentation of physicians' capacity and willingness to lead community-wide efforts to provide care to the medically underserved. The program also demonstrated the ability of communities to develop and run programs that suit their local needs. In assessing the program's accomplishments, Scott remains cautious. He notes that in 1993, as Reach Out began, about thirty-seven million people were without medical insurance, and the number swelled to forty-five million in 2005.

Realistically, the program was designed only to point the way to possible solutions; it could at best make only a modest dent in the uninsured problem. "A major expansion of Reach Out would not solve the growing problem of access to health care," he said. "One thousand organized programs, performing as the Reach Out projects have on average, would provide care to about five million uninsured and underserved persons—a small fraction of the large national problem."

Faith in Action (1992–2007, $86.5 million)

In 1992, the Foundation's board of trustees authorized the creation of its largest program to encourage volunteerism, Faith in Action. The program is designed to draw upon the spirit of helping others that is found in faith groups and to leverage it by providing funds to hire a full-time director at each site to organize and deploy volunteer services through an interfaith coalition. Local Faith in Action coalitions bring together volunteers from many faiths to work together to care for their neighbors with long-term chronic health needs.[10]

The volunteers, who come from churches, synagogues, mosques, and other houses of worship, provide services to their neighbors such as shopping for groceries, providing rides to doctors' appointments, cooking, and doing light housework. The most frequently provided services, in descending order, are friendly visitor–telephone reassurance (that is, keeping in touch with neighbors by phone, reminding them to take their medications, making sure that they have enough to eat, and simply checking in on them); transportation; meal preparation and delivery; linking people to community services; shopping; and respite for caregivers.

The majority of persons assisted by volunteers are old and very old women, homebound or unable to go out without help, poor or near poor, and living in isolation, with few social contacts. The Foundation re-authorized Faith in Action several times, but in 2005 decided not to renew it once its current funding ends, in 2007.

Improving Services for Homeless People

Health Care for the Homeless (1983–1990, $18 million);
Homeless Families Project (1989–1995, $5 million)

During the 1980s, homelessness took center stage as a largely unexpected new social problem. Homeless people have been found in most times and places, of course, but the increasing appearance of homeless women and children, and even whole families, on the streets and in shelters made the issue highly visible and compelling. Best estimates were that women and children totaled one-fifth to one-third of the homeless population. One heated debate at the time concerned the extent to which these families were homeless because of temporary economic dislocation or because of endemic poverty and other complicating factors.

The Foundation has made two large investments in national programs directed at alleviating problems facing homeless people in America. The first, Health Care for the Homeless, attempted to increase the availability of health care services for homeless people.[11] It became a model that was cited when the federal government passed the McKinney Act in 1987, providing federal dollars to improve access to health care for homeless people throughout the country.

The projects undertaken under the Health Care for the Homeless program, funded jointly with the Pew Charitable Trusts, were considered to be one of the single most effective networks of health care services developed for homeless people in the 1980s.[12] The creation of the program reflected the growth of the homeless problem and the fact that agencies that had historically been able to provide services to homeless people could no longer cope with their increasing numbers. Begun in 1983, the program was developed to provide cities—limited to the country's fifty largest—with an opportunity to make a significant impact on health care delivery to the homeless. Cosponsored by the U.S. Conference of Mayors, the program's guidelines required that cities forge a coalition of disparate groups of health care professionals and institutions, volunteer organizations, religious groups, public agencies, shelter providers, and members of the philanthropic community. These coalitions were charged with developing a program to meet the health care needs of the homeless, improving their access to other supportive services and entitlements, and conceiving a strategy for continuing the program services after the termination of foundation funding.

Nineteen cities participated in the program, each with a distinctly different approach based on its specific needs. In the early years of the program, service delivery methods included mobile vans outfitted as clinics, mobile teams going to existing programs that serve the homeless (particularly shelters and soup kitchens), and central clinics located in areas where homeless people could be found in substantial numbers.

After the Health Care for the Homeless program was completed, the Foundation funded a second program, the Homeless Families Program, which was more ambitious than its predecessor. It attempted to improve not only health care services for homeless families but also a range of other social services. The Foundation established a partnership with the U.S. Department of Housing and Urban Development, which made stable housing arrangements for families participating in the program.

The premise of the program was that both housing and social services (including health care) were needed to get many homeless families back into stable and independent lives. The Homeless Families Program exemplifies a range of national programs begun by the Foundation in the late 1980s and the start of the 1990s, which emphasized systems reform as a long-range solution to making social services more productive. The theory held that the problem with social services was not just that more were necessary but that existing resources needed to be better coordinated and better focused.

The Homeless Families Program was the first large-scale response to the problem of family homelessness. Started in nine cities across the nation, it had two complementary goals:

- To develop or restructure the systems of health, support services, and housing for families
- To develop a model of "services-enriched" housing for families that have multiple, complex problems

The ultimate goal of the program was to improve the residential stability of families, promote greater use of services, and increase steps toward self-sufficiency. Each of the nine sites received $600,000 in grants over five years to develop systems to care for homeless families and demonstrate a model of services-enriched housing for a group of families.

Corporation for Supportive Housing (1991–2000, $8 million); Taking Health Care Home (2002–2006, $6 million)

As much as 70 percent of the homeless population has health problems, mental and physical disabilities, and substance abuse problems. Supplying shelter to these individuals in the absence of health and supportive services is unlikely to result in their successful reintegration into society. Thus, the concept of "supportive housing" was born: permanent housing that combines health and social services for homeless people suffering from chronic health problems such as alcoholism, substance abuse, mental illness, and HIV/AIDS. Previous efforts to integrate access to health and social services with housing had been developed on a case-by-case basis, with no standard model for financing.

The Pew Charitable Trusts began this initiative with a feasibility study of a potential mechanism to promote the development of special-needs housing across the country. Pew brought together the Robert Wood Johnson Foundation's experience in special-needs housing and the Ford Foundation's experience in developing national financing for community-development programs to form a unique collaboration among three major philanthropic organizations that resulted in grants to create the Corporation for Supportive Housing.[13]

Early grants were used to select cities to test the feasibility of supportive housing, raise money to finance the housing from national, state, and local private and nonprivate sources, and provide technical assistance to community-based health and human services organizations and housing providers. Each community was required to match each dollar of the Corporation for Supportive Housing's national funding with one dollar of local philanthropic funding. In addition, states and localities committed capital and service funds to finance supportive housing development at each program site.

In 1995, grants from the Robert Wood Johnson Foundation, the Pew Charitable Trusts, and the Ford Foundation allowed the Corporation for Supportive Housing to establish programs at eight sites: New York City, Chicago, Columbus, Ohio, and the states of California, Connecticut, Michigan, Minnesota, and New Jersey. Through 1999, the Corporation for Supportive Housing raised more than $95 million from philanthropic and public funding sources. With this funding, it made grants and loans that backed the development of nearly 10,000 units of supportive housing, and leveraged more than $169 million in corporate investments to produce 4,000 more units.

The Foundation renewed its support of the Corporation for Supportive Housing with a $6 million, two-year program beginning in 2005 called Taking Health Care Home. Under the renewal, the existing eight supportive housing sites, plus two new ones, will receive funding, and a larger collaboration of foundations working to alleviate chronic homelessness will be established.

—ᴠᴠ— The Foundation and the Safety Net: An Assessment

For three decades, the Robert Wood Johnson Foundation and its leaders and staff have allocated hundreds of millions of dollars, countless hours of intellectual engagement, and incalculable well-intentioned effort into improving, stabilizing—or demonstrating the fragility of—the safety net. To hear past and present Foundation officers and grantees tell it, the Foundation deserves two cheers for its accomplishments.

"As far as doing work to make the safety net work better, they haven't made much of a mark," says John Billings, the NYU professor of health policy and a Foundation grantee. "They're beginning to take it on in a more head-on way, but historically they haven't." The Foundation's main downfall, Billings says, is its failure to recognize that an insurance card alone is not a panacea. "Of course coverage matters, and is the first and most important step," he says. "But a large share of the gap between rich and poor and different minority groups is how the providers are performing. A lot more time needs to be spent talking to patients about how they make health care decisions and where things go wrong. We tend to develop interventions based on what the middle class thinks is the right way, rather than recognizing the particular needs of these more vulnerable populations."

Steven Schroeder, former Foundation president and CEO, is equally blunt. "I don't think we have a very good feel for that," he says of safety net programs. "We came at these programs in different ways—by supporting workforce programs and by increasing Medicaid coverage for children, for example—but in terms of directly operating with safety net institutions, making grants accessible to them, I don't think we took it on frontally. I don't think we can look back and say that we directly helped the safety net institutions much, but I think we had a lot of programs that influenced them."

As Schroeder sees it, the Foundation could not agree on a clearly defined plan of attack. "I don't think we ever got a coherent strategy to bring to the board," he says. "The board was not the obstacle. You can frame it in one of two ways: We were not smart enough, or the task was too daunting for the resources we had. I suspect it was a mixture of both."

Paul Jellinek, who as a Foundation vice president played a key role in the shaping and implementing of several major safety net initiatives, takes a long view of the Foundation's safety net efforts. "The good news is that these programs were able to serve a fair number of people," he says. "The Foundation did make some headway in strengthening the financial viability of some community health centers; we did set up physician volunteer programs; Faith in Action set up hundreds of coalitions all over the country. But the bottom line is that we have forty-five million uninsured, and access to care is a huge problem for a lot of people. The argument is made that if we hadn't done what we did, the problem would be even worse. I'm not so sure about that."

Perhaps the last word belongs to the current Foundation president and CEO, Risa Lavizzo-Mourey. Calling the safety net "very much a priority," Lavizzo-Mourey says that the strategy going forward will focus on specific issues within vulnerable populations rather than on a generalized commitment to continue investing in the safety net.

> Safety net is a term that is not universally defined in the same way. Some people mean hospitals, some people mean hospitals and clinics. Some people mean federally qualified health centers, others place faith-based institutions in there—so it's a term that is difficult to get universal agreement on. However, many more people can agree on the populations, from a health care perspective, that are most vulnerable, most in need, most likely to have adverse outcomes or not realize their full health potential. So we look at it from that vantage point: who are the people in our society for whom the Robert Wood Johnson Foundation can make a difference? And how can we best go about doing so?

Notes

1. Institute of Medicine. *America's Health Care Safety Net: Intact but Endangered.* Washington, D.C.: National Academy of Sciences, 2000.
2. Fleming, G. V., and Anderson, R. M. "The Municipal Health Services Program: Improving Access While Controlling Costs?" Center for Health Administration Studies, Graduate School of Business and Division of Biological Sciences, University of Chicago, July 1984.
3. Ibid.
4. Finkler, S. A., and Hanson, K. L. "Innovations by Primary Care Health Centers: Lessons for Managers and Policy Makers." *Journal of Ambulatory Care Management,* 1995, *18*(2), 74–80.
5. Kovner, A. R. "The Hospital-based Rural Health Care Program: A Consortium Approach." *Hospital & Health Services Administration,* Fall, 1989, *34*, 3.
6. The Robert Wood Johnson Foundation, National Program Report on Communities in Charge. (www.communitiesincharge.org).
7. (http://www.dentalpipeline.org).
8. (http://www.urgentmatters.org/about/um_safety_net.htm).
9. Wielawski, I. M. "Reach Out: Physicians' Initiative to Expand Care to Underserved Americans." *To Improve Health and Health Care 1997: The Robert Wood Johnson Foundation Anthology.* San Francisco: Jossey-Bass, 1997. Available at (http://www.rwjf.org/reports/npreports/reachout.htm).
10. Jellinek, P., Gibbs Appel, T., and Keenan, T. "Faith in Action." *To Improve Health and Health Care 1998–1999: The Robert Wood Johnson Foundation Anthology.* San Francisco: Jossey-Bass. Available at (http://www.rwjf.org/reports/npreports/faithinaction.htm; http://www.fiavolunteers.org).

11. Rog, D. J., and Gutman, M. "The Homeless Families Program: A Summary of Key Findings." *To Improve Health and Health Care 1997: The Robert Wood Johnson Foundation Anthology.* San Francisco: Jossey-Bass, 1997. Available at (www.nhchc.org; www/bchhp.org).

12. "Homelessness, Health, and Human Needs." Washington, D.C.: The National Academy of Science, 1988.

13. (www.csh.org; http://www.rwjf.org/reports/grr/019309.htm).

Appendix. Safety Net Programs

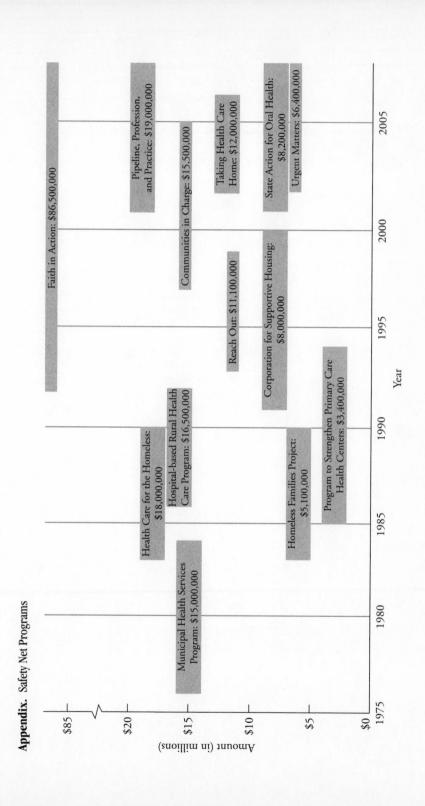

5

The Medicaid Managed Care Program

Marsha R. Gold, Justin S. White, and Erin Fries Taylor

Editors' Introduction

In the 1990s, as insurance companies and employers began to rely on managed care as a method for controlling health care costs, state governments followed suit by adopting managed care for their Medicaid programs. Medicaid pays for medical and long-term care for more than fifty million low-income Americans. It is financed by both the federal and state governments and is administered by the states. The task of adapting managed care to Medicaid was daunting, and in 1995 the Foundation developed an initiative—the Medicaid Managed Care Program—to help state governments, health plans, and consumers improve their use of managed care. The Foundation's staff felt that managed care represented an opportunity to both reduce the cost and improve the quality of health services delivered to low-income Americans.

      This chapter, written by the program's chief evaluator, Marsha R. Gold, and her colleagues at Mathematica Policy Research, describes the initiative and, drawing on the evaluation, offers an assessment of it. The authors discuss the various types of interventions used by the program to serve its constituencies, especially state governments and health plans. They also examine how the program, and the Center for Health Care Strategies where it is located, have evolved over the years.

Medicaid today is in crisis, devouring state budgets across the nation. Covering one out of every six Americans, the program costs $300 billion a year, having recently surpassed Medicare. It pays for some 60 percent of the nation's nursing home costs. In some states, Medicaid expenses, which have risen 63 percent in the past five years, account for a third of the budget. Even as the federal government threatens to reduce its contribution to the program, states are trying to find ways to slash their Medicaid budgets. Tennessee, for example, plans to cut off benefits for 320,000 Medicaid recipients in 2006.[1] Even though an initiative such as the Medicaid Managed Care Program doesn't address the root fiscal problems affecting Medicaid, its promise to help states buy higher-quality health services at lower cost and to assist health plans to provide better care for Medicaid patients bears careful watching.

---

1. Sara Lueck, "Surging Costs for Medicaid Ravage State, Federal Budgets." *Wall Street Journal,* Feb. 7, 2005, p. 1.

—ɯɯ— **M**edicaid, the main source of health insurance for a range of low-income, disabled, and seriously ill people, accounts for 17 percent of the nation's personal health spending.[1] More than fifty million people are enrolled in the program, including thirty-eight million low-income children and parents, and twelve million elderly and disabled people, half of whom also qualify for Medicare. The elderly and the disabled make up 25 percent of Medicaid beneficiaries but account for 70 percent of its spending. Although Medicaid is a national program, it is administered by the states; eligibility, benefits, and other program features vary substantially from state to state.

Enacted in 1965, Medicaid has been based largely on traditional fee-for-service insurance arrangements with health care providers; that is, providers willing to participate in the program were paid fees for the services they rendered. Starting in the 1970s, however, a few states experimented with offering Medicaid beneficiaries the option of enrolling in private managed care plans, especially health maintenance organizations, or HMOs.[2] For a monthly payment per person enrolled in the HMO (the "capitation rate"), the plans took responsibility for providing or arranging medical care covered under the state's program. States also pursued other managed care arrangements, such as primary care case management, which involves paying physicians a small monthly fee (in addition to fee-for-service) to coordinate care for their Medicaid patients.

In the 1990s, more states began to use managed care arrangements and to make enrollment in them mandatory for some categories of beneficiaries. Between 1990 and 1995, the percentage of Medicaid beneficiaries enrolled in managed care increased from 9 to 29 percent nationwide.[3] By 2003, some 60 percent of Medicaid beneficiaries nationwide were in managed care arrangements, primarily HMOs. Although states varied substantially in their use of managed care, thirty-four states and the District of Columbia had at least 25 percent of their Medicaid beneficiaries enrolled in HMOs in 2003 and nine had 75 percent or more. A higher percentage of children and families than disabled or elderly people were enrolled in HMOs.[4] Managed care remains a key part of Medicaid today in many states, even though some states experienced highly visible setbacks when health plans withdrew from their program, often because of conflicts over the adequacy of payment.[5]

Although state policymakers wanted to save money by moving Medicaid beneficiaries to managed care, they also hoped to improve the access to, and the quality of, care. In many states, the supply of physicians practicing in areas where Medicaid beneficiaries lived was limited, and the low fees that Medicaid paid to physicians restricted the number of those willing to participate in the program.[6] This led Medicaid enrollees to seek care in emergency rooms, hospital outpatient departments, and subsidized clinics instead of physicians' offices. Policymakers grew concerned that the lack of a medical provider to coordinate care would diminish the quality of services received by Medicaid beneficiaries and would ultimately lead to higher costs. They were particularly concerned about the quality of care for individuals with complex conditions—chronic illnesses, mental impairments, substance addictions—who required services from a range of providers.[7]

—⚍— The Medicaid Managed Care Program: History and Evolution

This environment of expanding Medicaid managed care and concern about quality spawned the Medicaid Managed Care Program, or MMCP, in the mid-1990s. Seeking to capitalize on the growing attention being given to Medicaid managed care, the Robert Wood Johnson Foundation established the MMCP in 1995 with the goal of improving access to and quality of care for Medicaid beneficiaries, particularly for those with chronic illness or disabilities.[8] (It reauthorized the program in 1999 and again in 2002. All told, the Foundation has committed $57 million to support the MMCP through mid-2006.) Led by a former Foundation staff member, Stephen Somers, the MMCP was housed in a new organization, the Center for Health Care Strategies, created especially to manage it.

Initial Program Structure

Initially, the Center for Health Care Strategies and the MMCP were essentially indistinguishable; the MMCP accounted for almost all the Center's funding. The MMCP's goals, profiled in its first call for proposals in 1996, were to assist states "in the design and evaluation of their Medicaid managed care policies" and assist health care providers and consumers in "the design, demonstration, and evaluation of new models of managed care for enrollees with chronic health and social problems." From the beginning, the MMCP awarded two main types of grants:

- *Model Demonstration Project Grants.* These grants provided up to $500,000 over a three-year period to support the development of new models to manage care for people with disabilities, chronic illness, and other complex care needs.[9] Typically awarded to states and health plans, the grants were intended to support innovative demonstration projects. In 1997, the program also authorized initial planning grants of up to $100,000. These enabled grantees to explore the feasibility of their proposal or to refine their plans before the MMCP decided whether to fund a full demonstration.

- *Best Practice or Policy Study Grants.* These grants provided up to $100,000 to state agencies, health plans, consumer organizations, health services researchers, and policy analysts. Best practice grants were awarded to identify, develop, and test innovative practices to improve the delivery of Medicaid managed care. Policy study grants documented best practices in management and operations of Medicaid managed care or provided analysis of market trends and policies that affect the implementation and outcomes of Medicaid managed care.

Between 1995 and 2002, twenty-five grants were awarded under the program for model development projects and 154 smaller grants for best practices or policy studies, though the former, by virtue of their size, accounted for a disproportionate amount of program spending. One early demonstration grant, awarded to the Delaware Department of Health and Social Services, went to developing a comprehensive Medicaid managed care model for elderly and physically disabled people and to designing a program that would provide managed long-term care for people with severe and persistent mental illness, substance abuse, or both. Under another model demonstration grant, the Washington Department of Social and Health Services selected Clark County to pilot a Medicaid managed care program for Supplemental Security Income recipients. As an example of an early best practice grant, the University of California, San Diego, produced a manual on risk-adjusted rate setting (that is, setting Medicaid payment schedules to providers that reflect the diagnosis and severity of illness of their patients). The chapter appendix provides examples of early model demonstration and best practice grants.

Both the Foundation and the Center for Health Care Strategies saw the model demonstration grants as particularly important, since they tested new methods of delivering care that could be shared broadly and help move the field. The Foundation gave the MMCP considerable discretion to make grants, including authority to make grants of up to $500,000 on its own. However, from the beginning, the MMCP found it difficult to attract strong proposals for model demonstration projects. Only twenty-six applications were received in response to the initial call for proposals in 1996, and only one of these was funded (though four additional proposals were awarded planning grants and three ultimately received funding for full-scale demonstrations).

As a consequence, in early 1997, the leadership of the Center for Health Care Strategies began to feel that the grantmaking strategy alone was not really an effective way to meet the program's objectives: the process was too passive, it relied on the strength of the applicants, and it generated weak proposals. Over the next few years, center staff members began to engage states more actively by focusing on assessments of their readiness for managed care and providing technical assistance.

Concurrently, the Foundation was addressing the same concerns as it considered whether to renew the grant. An internal Foundation assessment of the MMCP in late 1998 found that although the program had produced useful products and had earned respect as a neutral convener,

Medicaid managed care had progressed less rapidly than envisioned (particularly for the most vulnerable Medicaid beneficiaries—those with chronic illnesses and disabilities). The fact that most states' Medicaid managed care initiatives targeted families and children and not those qualifying for Medicaid because of their disabilities or chronic conditions—the initial focus of the MMCP—was proving to be a major limitation to the program model. The Foundation's analysis concluded that the MMCP could be strengthened with a more clearly defined and more effectively communicated and executed strategy.

Restructuring the Medicaid Managed Care Program

In reauthorizing the program for five years in 1999, the Robert Wood Johnson Foundation committed $13 million in additional funds for grants and, for the first time, $12 million for technical assistance. Under the new authorization, the MMCP shifted its priorities considerably.

- First, as a complement to making grants to states and others, it added an assistance strategy that involved primarily technical support. Over time, grant funds were increasingly linked to assistance and targeted in priority areas.

- Second, rather than targeting Medicaid managed care work to improve services for disabled and chronically ill Medicaid recipients, the MMCP focused more broadly on improving the quality of Medicaid managed care for all recipients by strengthening state governments' capacity to purchase quality services, by improving health plans' ability to measure and report on the quality of services, and, to a lesser extent, by helping consumers navigate the system.

Under the new approach, the MMCP can be viewed as helping state Medicaid programs and health plans pursue practices analogous to those of large private purchasers. The MMCP uses many of the same tools as others working on quality improvement—in particular, tools designed to help purchasers measure and reward good performance and encourage health plans to focus on quality. In the commercial sector, large employers lead the way, often requiring their managed care plans to be accredited by the National Committee for Quality Assurance, or NCQA. This requirement provides strong incentives for such plans to pursue quality improvement—incentives that are lacking for health plans that don't have an extensive commercial base, even though such plans have carved out a growing share of the Medicaid market. Since NCQA accreditation is expensive and typically geared to large employers, states rarely require it, but instead develop their own, somewhat parallel, series of quality improvement requirements for health plans in Medicaid.[10]

In 1999, the MMCP began to restructure its activities. It defined three core audiences—states, health plans, and consumers—and four core organizing principles around which its work would be structured:

- *Informed purchasing* to promote the purchasing of high-quality and cost-effective managed care services by states

- *Managed care best practices* to support quality improvements in clinical and administrative practices in managed care offered by participating health plans

- *Consumer action* to promote the ability of consumers to navigate health care delivery systems and to institutionalize a role for them in the design, implementation, and monitoring of publicly financed managed care

- *Integrated systems of care* to promote the integration of services and funding across public agencies, managed care organizations, and providers. (This was later dropped as a distinct element, because the Center for Health Care Strategies concluded that such concerns were relevant to all elements; the change allowed the MMCP to align its core principles with each of its core audiences.)

Most of the funding provided under the MMCP's reauthorization was used to develop initiatives built around each of the three main audiences identified by the Center for Health Care Strategies: the Purchasing Institutes for states; the Best Clinical and Administrative Practices, BCAP,

Initiative for health plans; and the Consumer Action Agenda for consumer groups.

- *Purchasing Institutes* are two- to three-day workshops that aim at helping Medicaid staff members improve their skills in buying health services through Medicaid managed care. Teams of senior staff members from different states attend. Institutes vary in focus and sophistication, but a basic one might include sessions on core skill areas like the basics of managed care purchasing; setting capitation rates; assessing the adequacy of provider networks; and monitoring access, quality, and performance. After each Institute, the participants are expected to return home and work to generate improvements in the areas covered at the Purchasing Institute. Since 2000, the MMCP has sponsored five basic Purchasing Institutes. Two additional Purchasing Institutes involving more intensive work over several meetings were convened specifically to help states monitor and reward managed care performance.

- *The Best Clinical and Administrative Practices Initiative* is designed to enhance the ability of Medicaid health plans to provide quality care within budgetary limits. Each BCAP work group involves staff members from ten to twelve health plans who get together in three or four structured meetings over nine to twelve months and work on improvements in a given clinical or administrative area, such as asthma or care for adults with chronic illness and disability. This is followed by an additional year of telephonic and other support from the Center for Health Care Strategies' staff. For example, work on asthma can involve developing registries of patients with asthmatic conditions, identifying those at particularly high risk, and doing outreach to help monitor and stabilize patients. The lessons from these groups are fed back to health plans in a variety of forms, including toolkits and meetings, such as the MMCP's periodic "Quality Summits," which are essentially interactive

conferences on quality issues for health plans. The MMCP
has held five BCAPs on improving birth outcomes, preventive care for children, asthma, children with special needs,
and adults with chronic illness and disability. The approach
is not unlike that of the Institute for Healthcare Improvement in its work with providers to improve care.[11]

- *The Consumer Action Agenda* aims at helping consumers
navigate and establish a formal role in Medicaid and similar
managed care systems. Small grants awarded to consumer
and family-based organizations have been the primary vehicle for advancing the Consumer Action Agenda. Two
rounds of grants have been awarded. In 2001, MMCP provided up to $25,000 each to nineteen grantees, and the
Robert Wood Johnson Foundation supplemented these
awards for ten grantees under its Covering Kids & Families
initiative. In 2002, the MMCP provided ten grants of
up to $50,000 each to consumer organizations represent-
ing people with disabilities and chronic illness. Activities
funded as part of consumer action grants include developing materials and convening educational seminars to help
consumers learn how to navigate Medicaid managed care;
training consumers in how to participate in the design or
monitoring of these systems; and developing peer support
services to allow consumers to help one another gain appropriate access to care.

The MMCP also convenes periodic meetings of the Managed Care
Solutions Forum (formerly called the Managed Care Pricing Forum) to
bring together stakeholders from all sectors to discuss emerging issues,
identify areas that need analysis, and provide feedback on reports, proposals, and policy initiatives. An early forum involved issues of setting
capitation rates and a later one involved issues associated with purchasing pharmaceuticals.

To provide an early assessment on the shift in strategy, the Robert
Wood Johnson Foundation asked Mathematica Policy Research to review
documents and interview participants in the programs. Mathematica's re-

port, submitted in 2001, found strong support for the programs from the MMCP's major constituencies, especially from Medicaid staff members who had the longest history with the Center for Health Care Strategies. Among all constituencies, the perception was that the MMCP was providing an important product that was not otherwise available. Particularly attractive to participants were the interactive forums and their focus on operations; they liked the fact that forums were focused on specific topics, strong in content, and small in scale. The report noted, however, that it was too soon to determine the ultimate effects of the new strategies and that future success would be likely to require developing a more integrated strategy that would create synergies among activities—grants and technical assistance, for instance.

Maturation and Diversification

Building on the Mathematica assessment, in 2001, the Robert Wood Johnson Foundation authorized $10 million in new funds to continue the program through June 2004, subsequently extended two years to December 2006. The new funds were integrated with about $20 million remaining from previous grants. Viewing grantmaking, technical assistance, and publications as related ways of achieving its goals, the MMCP gave priority in its grantmaking to states and health plans that participated in Purchasing Institutes or BCAP work groups. The Center for Health Care Strategies, which has the authority to vary the allocation of its MMCP funds between technical assistance and grants, over time has shifted more of its resources to the former. The MMCP has replaced its general grant solicitations with more targeted ones, aimed at those working with children with special needs, managed behavioral and general health care coordination, and managed long-term care, among others. Increasingly, the MMCP prefers small grants with substantial in-kind contributions.

As the MMCP has matured, it has sought to leverage the knowledge, respect, and products it had developed to attract other sources of financial support. For example, both the California HealthCare Foundation and the David and Lucile Packard Foundation have supported BCAP collaboratives in California and New York. This funding has allowed the

Center for Health Care Strategies to apply the BCAP approach in more settings and has also provided support to test out modifications to the model. In addition, the Center is developing a new Medicaid Disease Management Initiative, jointly funded by Kaiser Permanente and the Robert Wood Johnson Foundation, which focuses on improving care delivery for Medicaid recipients with multiple chronic conditions.

—⁓— What the MMCP Has Accomplished

In 2004, Mathematica completed a second evaluation of the MMCP— this time of the program as it operated between 2000 and 2003, a period when the MMCP was largely providing technical support to improve Medicaid managed care, with selected use of grants to support that objective. The MMCP might, for example, use grant funds to help states develop a measurement system that supports a new strategy developed in the Purchasing Institute; or it might invite a health plan with a grant that was focused on quality improvement in a given area to participate in a BCAP in the same area.

The evaluation distinguished the *reach* of the MMCP's activities from their *outcomes,* each of which is discussed below. Overall, the evaluation found that the program was reaching large sectors of its intended audiences with products that were well regarded, and that the support provided by the MMCP has led to concrete changes in the way some states and health plans deliver Medicaid managed care.

Program Reach, Participation, and Reputation

Reach defines the extent to which activities under the MMCP are known to the core audiences it seeks to help, the breadth and the intensity of participation by these audiences, and the opinions of core audiences on the quality and the value of the support they receive from the MMCP.

Information on these issues was gathered through surveys of the MMCP's core audiences, whether or not they participate in the program. Mathematica conducted telephone interviews with Medicaid directors in each state and surveyed key senior staff members involved in the states'

MMCP activities, the medical directors (or head of clinical quality) of all health plans participating in Medicaid nationwide, and a range of consumer groups with a potential interest in Medicaid managed care. It also identified and surveyed other stakeholders, including the staff involved in Medicaid managed care in the federal government (especially in the Centers for Medicare & Medicaid Services), public and private policy groups and associations, and the research community. The response rate was at least 85 percent for each group surveyed.

The survey findings were generally positive. The core audiences and stakeholders surveyed were typically aware of the Center for Health Care Strategies and its work on Medicaid managed care. Although the respondents also relied on other sources for information, they felt that the MMCP provided a unique resource that focused on operational concerns in ways that were unavailable elsewhere. For example, state Medicaid directors cited as strengths the Center's "connections and competence" and its "breadth of experience," its willingness "to try different things . . . to take risks and be demanding about what they [expect]," and its "institutional memory" and capacity for "being able to reach out . . . and dealing with all 50 states, or a majority of them, and knowing what works in one state and being able to translate that for other states." Health plans involved in BCAP appreciated the "hard-to-find forum that speaks to the particular challenges and issues of the Medicaid population."

By 2003, at least 75 percent of the states had participated in a Purchasing Institute, received a grant, or been the recipient of technical assistance. It was common for states to participate more than once and in multiple activities. Although health plans were a newer audience for the MMCP, about 42 percent of Medicaid managed care plans reported participating in one or more of the activities targeting them—BCAP work groups, one-time workshops or periodic quality summits, grants, and technical support activities. States and health plans overwhelmingly rated the activities in which they participated as excellent or good. In addition, awareness was high among other groups surveyed. However, this awareness was not necessarily deep; groups tended to be most aware of the activities targeted to them rather than of the full range of MMCP activities. Furthermore, health plans in which Medicaid made up a small share of total enrollment were less aware and less likely to participate in MMCP activities.

Outcomes Reflected in Changed Practices Among Core Audiences

Reputation is important, but a program's ultimate effectiveness must be judged by its outcomes. In this case, did the program make a difference in the way care is delivered under Medicaid managed care? For a complex and evolving program like the MMCP, this question is difficult to answer. To address it in this evaluation, Mathematica studied the experiences of the groups that most closely worked with the MMCP and examined overall trends.

States

The assessment of outcomes for the states built upon interviews with each Medicaid director in states with Medicaid managed care (forty-three of the forty-nine responded). Each responded to a set of questions about the MMCP's effect on the way they purchase Medicaid managed care. Half of those interviewed said they had made concrete improvements in their Medicaid managed care programs as a result of participating in MMCP, indicating that they saw the MMCP as fostering change and improvements in their programs. To get a better idea of the MMCP's impact, the evaluation then examined examples of changes reported by the states. Although some changes reported by directors involved hard-to-assess intangibles, such as providing ideas for new initiatives and validating state perceptions and strategies, we found evidence that at least ten states had made concrete, substantive improvements in their Medicaid managed care programs as a result of activities of, and interaction with, the MMCP (all but one remained in place as of fall 2004). Examples include the development and public reporting of health plan performance information, changes to the way states oversee quality in Medicaid managed care, and new ways of contracting and working with plans (see the box, Examples of MMCP's Work with States).

Examples of MMCP's Work with States

Maryland. Maryland worked to revamp what it viewed as an overregulated Medicaid managed care program. Drawing on its participation in multiple Purchasing Institutes and on-site technical assistance, the state evolved a "value-based purchasing strategy" and tools to support it. The intent of the strategy was to identify performance goals that could be monitored and a series of rewards that plans would get from meeting those goals. Maryland used administrative and survey data and dialogue with plans to develop eight performance measures and compliance indicators. It also developed a set of related incentive payments to reward providers who met standards. (The payments unfortunately could not be made, because the funds that had been reserved for them were taken out of Medicaid's budget.) With MMCP funds, Maryland tackled the issue of how to set rates by using risk-adjusted data by profiling plan performance. The state also developed a consumer report card to give visibility to high-quality plans.

Indiana. A new Medicaid director pushed her state—which she regarded as behind the field—to adopt some of the techniques that other states were using to purchase care under Medicaid. Through participation in a Purchasing Institute and on-site technical assistance, Indiana developed a managed care report card highlighting areas such as member satisfaction, quality of care, and access. Reactions were positive, and the report card is now being used annually. The Medicaid program also worked with local public health officials to bring a grassroots disease management program, which specifically targets those with diabetes, chronic heart failure, asthma, and hypertension, as well as those "at high risk of chronic disease," into the state's managed care program. Medicaid will fund chronic disease management as an extra benefit.

Michigan. The leadership of Michigan's Medicaid managed care program was concerned about the health plan choices available to beneficiaries and what the state paid to support these choices. Working with the MMCP, the Medicaid program incorporated quality-related and fiscal-solvency provisions into the bidding process. The changes led to a reduction in overall choice of health plans but an increase in the number of counties with more than one choice of plan. The changes also modified the way health plans were paid, and in so doing enhanced political support for the program.

As a complement to the Mathematica evaluation, the Robert Wood Johnson Foundation funded a separate study that included three state surveys to look for trends in their quality-monitoring activities.[12] These data provide strong evidence that states had substantially increased "value-based purchasing"—that is, looking for value while taking into account cost and quality—from 1995 to 2001. Generally speaking, states moved from viewing their role as primarily that of a bill payer to one involving more aggressive purchasing practices that sought value. Over this period, states were increasingly likely to collect data on enrollee satisfaction and access to and quality of health plans, make such data available to plans (and, to a lesser extent, enrollees), and develop targeted quality-improvement programs linked to these measures. Progress was uneven. For example, more progress was made in measuring satisfaction than in measuring quality. Within quality measurements more was done on childhood immunizations than on other areas; mental health and substance abuse were substantially less developed. While the MMCP cannot necessarily be credited with causing these changes, it is encouraging that the trend data show improvement in those areas in which the MMCP has been active.

Health Plans

The health plans surveyed also reported that MMCP participation led them to make changes in the way they deliver care. To confirm such reports, the evaluators conducted in-depth interviews with representatives of health plans that participated in four of the first five BCAP work groups. The majority of those interviewed said that the health plan had made changes as a result of the plan's participating in BCAP, with most of those changes still in place three to twelve months later and some plans continuing to generate change after the end of the BCAP. (See box, Examples of Changes in Care Delivery via BCAP.) Most participants said that BCAP had changed the way they think about quality improvement and had led them to approach the issue of quality differently in other clinical areas, not just in the BCAP's particular area of focus.

Examples of Changes in Care Delivery via BCAP*

Birth outcomes. One plan established an information hotline for pregnant women, gave them rewards if they reported pregnancies or completed postpartum visits, and developed a clinical outreach program to help follow up with members. In the first year of the program, identified pregnancies doubled and visit compliance increased 10 percent. The plan has now expanded the use of incentives to mammography and dental care. Another plan screens prenatal data, uses a risk assessment tool to conduct outreach, and has adopted new protocols to coordinate information and case management across the plan. The share of members with a completed risk assessment increased by 41 percent in the first five months.

Preventive care for children. One plan focused on improving early and periodic screening, diagnosis, and treatment, or EPSDT, rates for adolescents by providing incentives to both adolescent members and staff members at pilot community health centers. The plan increased the number of scheduled visits, and the EPSDT rate for adolescents at the sites increased by 12 percent over the first year of the pilot. The plan has since expanded the initiative statewide and has increased its overall EPSDT rate from 30 percent to 41 percent. Another plan increased its immunization

---

*Plan names are not used because the information was gathered on the promise of confidentiality.

rate for two-year-olds from 43 percent in 2000 to more than 60 percent in 2003 by educating providers about the importance of a reminder system and helping them adopt or improve their systems.

Asthma. One health plan developed an electronic asthma registry and uses it to sort children aged two to eighteen with asthma by their level of illness or risk. It uses an assessment survey to identify "out of control" asthmatics so that an action plan can be developed. The plan developed action plans for 63 percent of identified members before staff turnover stalled further progress. Another health plan developed a registry from multiple data sources, including data on health care claims over time. After identifying high-risk members, the plan offered providers a bonus for making changes to improve care management. Over twelve months, the physicians increased preventive asthma medication prescriptions by 6 percent, and emergency room use by asthmatics declined.

Adults with chronic illness. One health plan targeted disabled beneficiaries with congestive heart failure or diabetes and other comorbidities who resided in rural areas. Using a system of case management by telephone, the plan demonstrated a decline in hospitalization rates, length of stay, and total monthly costs per member that resulted in an overall 47 percent reduction in costs. The plan has since extended the telephonic case management intervention to other areas of the state. Another plan specializing in care for the disabled found that 70 percent of its members were at risk for three preventable conditions associated with immobility—pneumonia, urinary tract infection, and mechanical bowel obstruction. The plan taught members at risk for these conditions to notice and respond rapidly to symptoms and also educated primary care physicians on the same topic. The plan believed that the interventions improved care for two of the three preventable conditions, although developing adequate data on this point was difficult because of the small number of patients involved.

Whether the changes are having a positive effect is hard to know. Most health plans participating in BCAP struggled to track the outcomes of their interventions. Collecting process measures of change proved harder for some topics, such as chronic disease in adults and birth outcomes, than for others, such as asthma and preventive care for children, largely because the latter have a strong evidence base on which to structure interventions and accepted measures of performance. Health plans that made little progress under BCAP or terminated their efforts early tended to be ones that experienced turnover in leadership or staff, or both, or adverse financial circumstances. Organizational stability appears to be an important precondition to maintaining improvements in care. Thus, states seeking to improve Medicaid managed care will benefit by encouraging as much stability as possible in the plans that participate in Medicaid managed care.

Consumer Groups

To help consumers navigate and interact with Medicaid managed care, the MMCP made two rounds of grants ranging from $25,000 to $50,000. These grants funded activities such as developing materials and holding education sessions, arranging meetings to involve consumers in the policy process or teach them how to get involved, and creating peer support programs to facilitate access to health care services. Although grantees typically did what they had proposed to do, the grants tended to be too few, too small, too localized, and too short in duration to lead to sustainable or broad-based change. Despite the lack of success, consumer groups viewed this support as important and were disappointed that more grant funding was not forthcoming.

Overall Program Effectiveness

The evaluation concluded that although there was room for improvement, the Medicaid Managed Care Program was effective in working with two of its three core audiences (states and health plans) during the period examined—2000 to 2003; it had less success in helping consumers, the third of its three target audiences. The MMCP's integration of technical assistance with other support to state Medicaid agencies and Medicaid managed care plans appears to have led many staff members of these organizations to change their thinking about the way they purchase and provide Medicaid managed care. In a meaningful number of cases, they viewed the combination of technical assistance and grants as more effective than either one alone. This was truer for the states, which had more grant experience with the MMCP, than health plans. Moreover, the MMCP has allowed the Center for Health Care Strategies to mature and gain respect, generating support and capacity that can be tapped by the Robert Wood Johnson Foundation and other foundations to pursue related program goals.

There are areas where performance could be stronger. In a field where leadership turns over frequently, the MMCP has not been as aggressive as it might have been in working with newly appointed state officials. In addition, although measurement is a crucial component of quality improvement, health plans participating in BCAP still struggle to develop valid measures to judge performance. The MMCP's reach is also much stronger for Medicaid-dominant plans than for commercial plans in which Medicaid makes up only a small share of enrollment. The MMCP's focus on consumers, its third core audience, has also been limited. Although many consumer groups are aware of the MMCP, the program has invested relatively little in initiatives to strengthen them.

—⁓— Insights on Broader Issues

Beyond these findings, the MMCP evaluation sheds light on a number of issues facing philanthropies that pursue social change. These issues include the challenges in creating sustainable and meaningful change; whether support for change should target high, average, or low performers; and who should and will support efforts needed to build the infrastructure that an emphasis on prudent purchasing and quality improvement requires.

Creating Sustainable Change

A key question is how to support efforts that lead to valuable and sustainable change rather than those that leave little mark. Exploring the factors within the MMCP that facilitated or impeded meaningful change can provide some guidance in answering this question.

The MMCP experience suggests that its operational and hands-on support was helpful to states and health plans. Furthermore, the program's group-based support—through Purchasing Institutes and workshops that generated interaction among states and plans—leveraged resources and was viewed by participants as important. There also seems to be a relationship between the intensity of MMCP assistance received and successful change.

The MMCP evaluation also indicates that the commitment of top leaders within the organizations is important. Turnover in leadership can undercut progress, but sustainability can be achieved if change can be institutionalized within a program. Under the MMCP, it often took a new director or a crisis to generate interest and the support needed to change the way Medicaid managed care was purchased. As many as one-quarter of all state Medicaid directors can turn over in a year, as they did between 2003 and 2004. If a change becomes part of the institution before new staff members arrive, the new people might simply accept the change as a normal part of the program.

Rapid turnover of state health officials, however, makes it hard to maintain the commitments needed to sustain change. In health plans, turnover may be an even more important barrier. In plans, quality could sometimes be improved "under the radar screen" by a dedicated medical director, but unless it had the support of the health plan's leadership, it often died when the medical director left. Stability—both in the overall state program in which health plans operate and in the fiscal and organizational context of their own organization—is also important to the ability of health plans to introduce change.

Constraints of the Macro-Environment

The most fundamental threat to the success of programs like the MMCP is the eroded economy in many states and in the nation—a factor cited by all stakeholders as the primary constraint in all their efforts to improve Medicaid managed care. With fiscal stringency, managed care appears unlikely to disappear. Indeed, many state government officials look to the MMCP to help them become more efficient in negotiating the difficult economic environment. Tight resources, however, make it more challenging to keep plans and providers affiliated with the program, and change is hard to introduce if programs are unstable.[13] Fiscal stringency also puts a premium on cost-saving innovation. Though tight budgets generate interest in more prudent purchasing of Medicaid managed care, they also can generate unrealistic expectations about what kind of cost savings Medicaid managed care can deliver and how fast.

Medicaid's complex layers of eligibility reflect the use of the program by policymakers to provide a safety net and address coverage concerns and multiple unmet health care needs in our country.[14] Increased enrollment, including coverage of some people with very expensive needs, adds to Medicaid's costs and strains the Medicaid budget. To the extent that the federal government and state governments reduce funding for Medicaid managed care, it will be harder for states to maintain the participation of health plans and providers and improve quality of care.

Targeting an Audience: Working with Leaders Versus Followers

Programs like the MMCP typically face tensions in defining their target audience. Working with "stars" can increase the probability of success and can serve to lead the field, but these high-performers might have succeeded on their own. Focusing on them may leave the rest of the field behind. The MMCP staff may like to target leading states capable of cutting-edge strategies that can then influence other states. But in fact the states that the MMCP works with are quite varied in the sophistication of their Medicaid managed care purchasing. Although participation was highest for the most sophisticated states (as judged independently by experts and surveys of state purchasing practices), participation levels were high among all but the least sophisticated states. Furthermore, states with both high-level and moderate-level sophistication made concrete changes as a result of the program. Indeed, by some measures, moderately sophisticated states showed as much success as the most sophisticated ones, sometimes more.

Building Infrastructure: Whose Job Is It?

Changing purchasing practices and the way care is delivered requires substantial investment. It takes time and money to build the understanding, skills, and technical infrastructure to buy care well and to deliver a quality product. Foundations often are called upon to weigh the value of investing in infrastructure development, whose benefits are long-term and sometimes difficult to quantify, against investing in short-term projects whose value can be assessed more rapidly and in more tangible ways. Many foundations are reluctant to fund the former. The MMCP experience indicates, however, that outside support that complements internal organizational resources is valuable as a way of encouraging change, conveying technical insights, and developing the infrastructure essential to high-quality Medicaid managed care programs.

One can make the case that the ultimate responsibility for funding the kind of support provided by the MMCP lies with the entities responsible for the Medicaid program: the federal and state governments. But federal policy increasingly positions Medicaid as a state responsibility, and as a result technical assistance by federal agencies has diminished. Both state governments and health plans face substantial barriers in generating funds and resources for the kind of quick-turnaround support and training that the MMCP provides.[15] In any case, a centralized focus is likely to be important in helping states and plans learn from one another. In this context, stakeholders may look to philanthropy to fill gaps.

—ɯ— The Bottom Line

In 1975, Howard H. Hiatt M.D., then dean of the Harvard School of Public Health, wrote an influential article on "Protecting the Medical Commons: Who Is Responsible?"[16] He likened the challenges in health care to those of shepherds sharing a field. With limited resources (a single field), there are trade-offs between the individual and collective good. Although Hiatt's focus was on medical technology and the decisions physicians make about who gets what, the tensions he described parallel those inherent in building an infrastructure for quality improvement. Though all seek its benefits, the incentives of the current structure do not yield the investments needed to generate them. This is a problem if policymakers are serious about the importance of leveraging purchasing to pursue better-quality care.

It is one thing to set a goal for improving Medicaid managed care. It is quite another to accomplish that goal when Medicaid exists in an environment of limited funds and support. The MMCP highlights the contribution that day-to-day work by states and health plans can make in improving care under Medicaid managed care. But on-the-ground efforts can be successful and maintained only to the extent that Medicaid itself is able to generate adequate and continuing support for quality improvement and for the program itself.

Appendix: Examples of Early MMCP Grantmaking, 1996–1998

Model Demonstration Grants	Award Date
A Strategy to Provide Medicaid Managed Care Services to the Disabled (Commonwealth of Massachusetts)	June 1996
Study of Mental Health Crisis Intervention Services for Dually Eligible Elderly (Mt. Hood Community Mental Health Center, Oregon)	October 1996
Innovative Efforts to Integrate and Restructure Managed Care to the Medically Indigent (University Health System, Texas)	January 1997
Development of an Integrated System of Health and Support Services for SSI Beneficiaries (Clark County, Washington)	January 1997
Integration of Services for Children with Mental Health Needs (Greater Kansas City Community Foundation, Missouri)	August 1997
Development of Criteria for Medicaid Managed Care Special Needs Plan (County of Chemung, New York)	October 1997
A System of Managed Care for Persons with Serious Mental Illness and Substance Abuse (State of Wisconsin)	February 1998
Medicaid Managed Care for Special Needs Populations (State of Utah)	April 1998
Healthier Babies Project (Health Partners, Pennsylvania)	April 1998
Development and Implementation of AIDS Centers of Excellence (Tennessee Opportunity Programs Inc, Tennessee)	July 1998
The Safety Net Project (State of Colorado)	September 1998
Implementation of Statewide Managed Long-Term Care in Delaware (State of Delaware)	December 1998

Best Practice Grants	Award Date
Consumer Participation in Developing and Monitoring Medicaid Managed Care (National Health Law Program, North Carolina)	January 1996
Rate Setting for High-Risk Populations (Regents of the University of California for work with 11 states)	March 1996
Member Satisfaction Survey with Acute Care AHCCCS Medicaid Managed Care (Arizona Health Care Cost Containment System)	March 1996
Data Requirements in Medicaid Managed Care (The MEDSTAT Group, Illinois)	July 1996
Conference on Current Approaches for Medicaid Client Education (Center for Health Policy Development, Maine)	August 1996
A Health Status Based Method for Risk-Adjusted SSI Premiums (University of Washington, Washington)	August 1996
Conference on Alternative Managed Long-Term Care Models for CA (The MEDSTAT Group, California)	April 1998
Case Management in Medicaid Managed Care for People with Developmental Disabilities (Developmental Disabilities Health Alliance)	July 1998

Notes

1. Kaiser Commission on Medicaid and the Uninsured. *The Medicaid Program at a Glance.* Washington, D.C.: Kaiser Family Foundation, January 2004.

2. Spitz, B. "Contracting with Health Maintenance Organizations." In R. J. Blendon and T. W. Moloney (eds.), *New Approaches to the Medicaid Crisis.* New York: F&S Press, 1982, pp. 177–197.

3. Kaiser Family Foundation. State Health Facts On-Line, Selected Tables on Medicaid Managed Care and Trends. (www.statehealthfacts.org), accessed Oct. 25, 2004.

4. Schneider, E. C., Landon, B. E., Tobias, C., and Epstein, A. M. "Quality Oversight in Medicaid Primary Care Case Management Programs." *Health Affairs,* Nov.-Dec. 2004, *23*(6), 235–242.

5. Draper, D. A., Hurley, R. E., and Short, A. C. "Medicaid Managed Care: The Last Bastion of the HMO?" *Health Affairs,* 2004, *23*(2), 155–167.

6. See, for example, Gold, M., Mittler, J., Draper, D., and Rosseau, D. "Participation of Plans and Providers in Medicaid and SCHIP Managed Care." *Health Affairs,* Jan.-Feb. 2003, *22*(1), 77–88; Zuckerman, S., McFeeters, J., Cunningham, P., and Nichols, L. "Changes in Medicaid Physician Fees, 1998–2003: Implications for Physician Participation." *Health Affairs,* June 23, 2004, *W4–374*; and Bindman, A., Yoon, J., and Grumback, K. "Trends in Physician Participation in Medicaid: The California Experience." *Journal of Ambulatory Care Management,* 2003, *26*(4), 334–343.

7. Vladeck, B. "Where the Action Really Is: Medicaid and the Disabled." *Health Affairs,* Jan.-Feb. 2003, *22*(1), 62–76; Frank, R. G., Goldman, H. H., and Hogan, M. "Medicaid and Mental Health: Be Careful What You Ask For." *Health Affairs,* Jan.-Feb. 2003, *22*(1), 101–113; and Crowley, J. S., and Elias, R. *Medicaid's Role for People with Disabilities.* Washington D.C.: Kaiser Family Foundation, Aug. 2003.

8. For additional information describing the program, see White, J. S., and Gold, M. *The Medicaid Managed Care Program of the Center for Health Care Strategies.* Washington, D.C.: Mathematica Policy Research, Dec. 2004. (Available from the Robert Wood Johnson Foundation.)

9. The maximum funding level was increased to $750,000 in 2002, but grants of this size are rare.

10. Felt-Lisk, S. "Monitoring Quality in Medicaid Managed Care: Accomplishments and Challenges at Year 2000." *Journal of Urban Health: Bulletin of New York Academy of Medicine,* Dec. 2000, *77*(4), 536–559.

11. Berwick, D. M. "Developing and Testing Changes in Healthcare Delivery." *Annals of Internal Medicine,* Apr. 15, 1998, *128*(8), 651–565; Kilo, C. M. "A Framework for Collaborative Improvement: Lessons from the Institute for Healthcare Improvement's Breakthrough Series." *Quality Management in Health Care,* 1998, *6*(4), 1–13,.

12. Landon, B. E., Schneider, C. T., and Epstein, A. "The Evaluation of Quality Management in Medicaid Managed Care." *Health Affairs,* July-Aug. 2004, *23*(4), 245–254,.

13. Gold, Mittler, Draper, and Rosseau (2003).

14. Rowland, D., and Tallon, J. R. "Medicaid: Lessons from a Decade." *Health Affairs,* Jan-Feb. 2003, *22*(1), 138–144; and Holahan, J., and Ghosh, A. "Understanding the Recent Growth in Medicaid Spending, 2000–2003." *Health Affairs,* Jan. 2005, *W5–52*.

15. White and Gold (2004); and Martin, R., and Kenneson, M. "A Focused Survey of the Medicare and Medicare Payor Markets for Convening and Programmatic Technical Assistance." Submitted to the Robert Wood Johnson Foundation by Mathematica Policy Research on August 25, 2004. The latter identified a number of barriers to state support for such activities. These barriers include difficulties in securing relatively small dollar amounts for staff training and educational activities, budget and administrative constraints on staff travel, and lack of capacity for developing effective proposals to secure outside foundation funds, which limit interest in seeking support for small amounts of money that do not justify the effort. Martin and Kenneson also found that federal funding for Medicaid technical assistance has diminished over time, since federal policy regards this form of support as a state responsibility. Though health plans may have more administrative flexibility, they tend to rely on monthly capitation financing streams that are both tight and poorly suited to generating large amounts of capital for investments.

16. *New England Journal of Medicine,* 1975, *293,* 135–140.

6

The Evolution of the Robert Wood Johnson Foundation's Approach to Alcohol and Drug Addiction

Victor A. Capoccia[1]

Editors' Introduction

This chapter by Victor Capoccia, a senior program officer at the Robert Wood Johnson Foundation and head of the team that shapes its grantmaking in preventing and treating alcohol and drug addiction, offers an inside look at the Foundation's strategies that have shaped its billion-plus dollars in investments to reduce the harm caused by alcohol and drug misuse in America. One of a number of *Anthology* chapters that examine how the Foundation has addressed prevention and treatment of drug and alcohol addiction,[1] it sets the Foundation's work into the context of national policy and traces its evolution since its first grants in the 1980s.

    The public perception and the politics of addiction prevention and treatment have been shaped by a cultural war over the reasons for substance abuse. Whether addiction is viewed as a criminal problem, a moral failing, a social problem, or a chronic health care condition (and it has been seen as all of these) will influence the approaches to addressing it. These can range from the incarceration of drug users to self-help programs such as Alcoholics Anonymous and from community-based prevention programs to medical treatment.

As Capoccia observes, the Foundation, influenced by recent scientific knowledge about the biological and neurological causes of addiction, considers addiction to be a chronic health condition. As such, it should be treated like other chronic conditions. Capoccia also makes it clear that, given the scientific evidence that some people are going to become addicted no matter what is done to prevent addiction, prevention efforts alone will not solve the problem; an approach combining both prevention and treatment is needed.

1. The author would like to thank Kristin Schubert and Emily Day for their research assistance and Molly McKaughan for identifying reports on past grants.
2. Hughes, R. G. "Adopting the Substance Abuse Goal: A Story of Philanthropic Decision Making." In *Anthology 1998–1999* (1998); Mangione, T., Howland, J., and Lee, M. "Alcohol and Work: Results from a Corporate Drinking Study." In *Anthology 1998–1999* (1998); Diehl, D. "Recovery High School." In *Anthology, Vol. V* (2002); Brodeur, P. "Combating Alcohol Abuse in Northwestern New Mexico: Gallup's Fighting Back and Healthy Nations Programs." In *Anthology, Vol. VI* (2003); Wielawski, I. M. "The Fighting Back Program." In *Anthology, Vol. VII* (2004); Jellinek, P., and Schapiro, R. "Join Together and CADCA: Backing Up the Front Line." In *Anthology, Vol. VII* (2004); Parker, S. G. "Reducing Youth Drinking: The 'A Matter of Degree' and 'Reducing Underage Drinking Through Coalitions' Programs." In *Anthology, Vol. VIII* (2005); Chapter Six in this volume.

—w— ew fields have felt the ages-old clash between belief and science more acutely than that of alcohol and drug dependence. Over the past half century—and in the last ten years in particular—science has made great strides in understanding the nature of addiction and how it can be treated. Addiction research has demonstrated that alcohol or drug misuse alters the brain's natural patterns for satisfaction and gratification; that dependence on alcohol and drugs is treatable; and that the harmful effects of alcohol and drug abuse on young people can be reduced by making it more difficult for them to acquire alcohol and drugs. What's more, recent science has led to the view that the misuse of alcohol and drugs is not only a public health issue but also an issue of personal health. In other words, such misuse has come to be seen as a chronic illness—one that requires new policy and new programmatic responses.

Even so, alcohol abuse and drug dependence are still often not recognized as chronic illnesses or treated as such. And although treatment for these conditions is known to be as effective as treatment for asthma, diabetes, and other chronic illnesses, the nation's health system generally does not recognize and treat the condition. When it does, it is set up to treat only 20 percent of the need. And that need is great. Nearly one in ten Americans over the age of twelve has a problem with alcohol or drugs—some 22 million people in all.[1] Alcohol and drugs have been estimated to be the cause of more than 144,000 deaths a year and 20 percent of the nation's hospital costs.[2, 3] They are also a significant factor in child welfare cases and family problems.

Given the enormous personal and social costs that could be avoided by preventing and treating alcohol and drug dependence, why isn't more being done? One answer is that in the formation of public opinion and public policy, belief has trumped science. In other words, despite the advances in scientific research, despite a substantial body of empirical evidence to the contrary, much of the public still believes that the abuse of alcohol and drugs is a willful act—essentially a personal, moral failing. Unfortunately, this belief does not acknowledge the recent scientific research that has shown alcohol and drug dependence to derive from a powerful confluence of biological, social, and environmental factors that also form the basis of other chronic illnesses.

From the time it was established as a national philanthropy, in 1972, the Robert Wood Johnson Foundation has invested more than a billion dollars on programs to combat the harmful effects of alcohol and drugs, and in that time its programs have gone through three stages. These stages have reflected the struggle within society and within the Foundation of three ways of viewing alcohol and drug misuse: first, that it is primarily a social issue—rather than a health issue—that leads to crime and community disintegration; second, that it is largely a matter of behaviors deeply rooted in complex societal norms that can be affected by interventions that modify behavior or reduce access to the substances; and third, that it is a health issue involving a preventable and treatable chronic condition.

—w— Phase I: Help for Alcoholics

Although Robert Wood Johnson, in his personal philanthropy, had an interest in helping, in his words, "men with drinking problems," in its very earliest days the foundation named after him had at best a passing interest in the issue of alcohol misuse. The Robert Wood Johnson Foundation's first formal involvement began in 1982 with a staff proposal to the board of directors suggesting a Foundation initiative to help address the problems of alcohol-related illness.

The proposal was stimulated by a 1980 Institute of Medicine report, *Alcoholism, Alcohol Abuse, and Related Problems: Opportunities for Research,* which provided the first comprehensive review of research on alcohol use and abuse and called for increased research on the topic. According to Robert Blendon, who was a Foundation senior vice president at the time and is currently a professor at the Harvard School of Public Health, the proposal was developed because the costs to society and to the health care system were significant, and there was a great need to know more about misuse and how to treat it.

The 1982 proposal demonstrated a clear understanding of the excessive use of alcohol as a health condition as well as a major social problem. It noted that despite the tremendous cost that alcoholism and alcohol abuse imposed on society, 85 percent of problem drinkers and alcoholics received no treatment for their condition. Furthermore, it reported that the gap between the numbers of those who needed treatment and those who received it existed for three reasons: societal ambivalence about whether alcoholism was a disease or more of a moral issue; a lack of information about which methods were effective in treating the condition; and society's unwillingness to pay for treatment. The proposal concluded with a call for the staff to encourage individual proposals that would seek to evaluate the cost-effectiveness of specific treatments for alcohol-related health problems, and their applicability in different settings. This recommendation marked the first step in developing the Foundation's understanding of alcoholism not as a social problem but as a medical condition with social implications.

The board ultimately turned down the staff proposal, largely because it ran counter to a policy that avoided disease-specific, or condition-focused, investments. But in 1983 the Foundation did award a one-year $57,000 grant to Boston University for the first phase of a study on alcoholism treatment in industry. (The full study was eventually supported by National Institute of Alcoholism and Alcohol Abuse.) The project was justified as part of a Foundation initiative on cost containment and health services research. This study, which involved employees of a large aircraft engine plant, compared the costs and outcomes of alcohol-abuse treatment offered at an inpatient hospital versus treatment offered through employee assistance or self-help programs.[4]

While the 1982 staff proposal was noteworthy for its focus on alcoholism as a treatable health condition, it did not touch on three issues that later emerged as the Foundation's strategic priorities: reducing underage drinking; preventing excessive alcohol use; and curbing drug use. These issues were not unknown at the time. According to a national survey on drug abuse in 1979, some 50 percent of young people from ages twelve to seventeen reported alcohol use in the preceding month.[5] Data collected annually since 1975 have shown that nearly 80 percent of young people eighteen and under have consumed alcohol by the time they reach the twelfth grade, and that 12 percent of eighth-graders have consumed five or more drinks on a single occasion in the two weeks preceding the survey.[6]

The omission of drug use from the Foundation's priorities was surprising, given the political environment of the period. At that time, considerable attention was given to the problem of drug abuse, in part through Nancy Reagan's Just Say No campaign and in part through television ads showing drug-abused brains as eggs in a frying pan. Society viewed drug use more as a social and criminal issue than as a health issue. Harsh penalties for possessing and selling drugs appeared in new state and federal laws. Most federal, state, and local funding was directed toward interdiction of drugs. No person running for political office could risk being soft on crime or sympathetic to drug users. Moreover, at the time, there was only the beginning of an academic, governmental, and treatment infrastructure that focused on illegal drug use, and it was distinct from the infrastructure concerned with alcohol. In the early 1980s, states typically had an office of alcohol services within their public health structure, and several offices concerned with drugs within public safety and mental health agencies. Thus, at the time, it was easy for the Foundation to view drugs as primarily a social problem that was outside the purview of an organization devoted to health and health care.

—⚒— Phase II: Recognition of Drugs and Tobacco Use and Focus on Underage Alcohol Use

By the middle and later 1980s, even though the prevalence of drug use had remained relatively stable, social and political conditions and the kinds of drugs that were widely available had changed since the early years of the decade, leading to a shift in the federal government's policy focus. The changes can be seen in three events.

1. The death of Len Bias in 1986 from a cocaine overdose forced a nation that had overlooked the growth of cocaine and crack use to confront this reality. Bias played basketball at the University of Maryland, was an All-American, and was a first-round draft choice of the Boston Celtics. He died less than forty-eight hours after being drafted. More than any other single factor, Bias's death prompted

the media to take a hard look at the extent and the costs of cocaine use.

2. An influential national movement of middle-class parents concerned about their children's use of marijuana developed.[7] The parents' movement exercised political influence beyond its numbers by dint of perseverance, belief, and focused communications about the threat of casual drug use. The voices of concerned parents found a receptive ear in first lady Nancy Reagan, who adopted the prevention of illicit drug use as her special project. The issue of drug use among young Americans was framed as part of a "culture war" and a threat to values. Clearly, the parents' movement did not define drug use as a health issue, and apparently never viewed underage alcohol use as a similar threat.

3. The government's response to the strong public concern over drug use was crystallized in Congress's establishing the Office of National Drug Control Policy in 1988 to coordinate drug policy in the United States, with Cabinet-level authority in the Office of the President. President George H. W. Bush appointed William Bennett, who brought previous Cabinet-level experience as President Reagan's Secretary of Education, and certifiable conservative credentials, to the position of the nation's first drug czar. Bennett used the office to foster his belief that drug use was a deviant behavior, reflecting moral breakdown. Throughout this period, the Office of National Drug Control Policy did not consider the drug problem as a health issue.

In this political and social climate, the Robert Wood Johnson Foundation responded with two overlapping efforts. The first began in 1986 with a staff report that presented strategies for addressing the problems of "substance abuse" and dependence. The second began in 1991 with a staff report that led to board approval of three goal areas, including substance abuse, and presented a comprehensive framework for the Foundation's work in the alcohol and drug field.

The 1986 Staff Report and Its Implications

The 1986 staff report summarized recent opinion polls that documented society's view of and concern with widespread drug use, and emphasized the cost and mortality associated with alcohol and drug misuse. It recommended that the Foundation support two or three institutions with active treatment programs and a strong interest in prevention, which would be demonstrated through a wide range of activities, including genetic and epidemiological studies, improved methods of treatment matching, testing of new treatment models, evaluation of treatment and prevention programs, and training clinical researchers as well as community service providers.

Two years later, the Foundation developed its first major program to address substance abuse—one that took an approach different from that proposed in the 1986 staff report. In July 1988, the board approved a $26 million program to support community initiatives to reduce the demand for illegal drugs and alcohol, which became known as Fighting Back.[8] The Foundation eventually invested $88 million over fifteen years to demonstrate and evaluate the benefits of this approach. Fighting Back was based on the idea that if the right combination of leaders in a community worked together in a coalition to address drugs and alcohol, the threat that these represented to neighborhoods could be significantly reduced, if not eradicated.

The 1986 staff report and the Fighting Back program departed from the orientation of phase one in three ways.

- The Foundation not only recognized the issue of problem drug use but also came to regard drugs and alcohol as a single problem area. This connection was significant in a nation that had separated funding, regulation, research, and treatment systems for each substance.
- The Foundation, which was comfortable supporting specific program interventions, such as halfway houses, school-based health clinics, and health care for homeless persons, was now willing to fund a community process that might or

might not lead to program interventions. This was not a classic health approach to a medical condition.

- The Foundation explicitly supported a program that focused on mitigating the social dimensions of a health issue. Coalitions were to concentrate on increasing public awareness, promoting activities for young people that kept them away from drugs and alcohol, reducing crime, reducing work-related absence and accidents, improving neighborhoods, and screening for alcohol and drug problems.

The Partnership for a Drug-Free America was another initiative that received funding in the late 1980s. Created by Phil Joanou, a former advertising executive who recognized the potential of communications and marketing as a tool to discourage the demand for drugs, the Partnership enlisted major advertising agencies to volunteer their creative talent and resources to produce anti-drug advertisements. Often, the federal government provided the funds that paid for ads on television and radio and in print media.

The 1991 Goal Report and Its Programmatic Implications

By 1991, the Foundation was deeply involved in the issue of alcohol and drugs through the Fighting Back program—an approach that the federal government replicated by allocating more than $300 million to support some 251 coalitions in forty-five states in a program called the Community Partnership Demonstration Grant Program. And 1991 also marked the first year of Steven Schroeder's twelve-year tenure as president of the Foundation. In his interview with the trustees when he was a candidate for the Foundation's presidency, Schroeder stressed the harm caused by alcohol, drugs, and tobacco, and promised to devote some of the Foundation's resources to addressing this issue. This was especially appealing to James Burke, then a member of the Foundation's board, who also served on the board of directors of the Partnership for a Drug-Free America and was chairman of the President's Drug Advisory Council.

In 1991, the Foundation's board approved three broad goal areas, one of them having to do with alcohol and drugs. These were the goals:

- To assure access to basic health care

- To improve the way services are organized and provided to people with chronic health conditions

- To reduce the harm caused by "substance abuse," including tobacco, alcohol, and "illicit" drugs

The discussion about whether to make "substance abuse" a formal goal of the Foundation was guided by a 1991 staff report that cited both the alarming use of alcohol, tobacco, and drugs, especially among young people, and the social and health-related costs of what was then considered to be a problem of epidemic proportions. The report zeroed in on two dimensions not seen in earlier work: tobacco as a substance of concern, and patterns of alcohol and tobacco use among young people as a target of concern. The report offered two overarching strategies to guide the Foundation's future work: (1) improving the understanding of the causes of substance abuse, and (2) expanding the understanding of problem alcohol and drug use and the capacity for delivering effective interventions. The report offered a broad societal perspective as a context for alcohol and drug use: "We are confronted with a problem affecting all segments of our society, one that has effects far beyond the immediate health risks associated with the use and abuse of substance." The board accepted this broad perspective and avoided language that would imply personal responsibility for the misuse of alcohol and drugs.

An initiative to reduce substance abuse among Native Americans, known as Healthy Nations, followed the goal report. Authorized in 1991 Healthy Nations provided technical assistance and grants to Native American governmental and not-for-profit organizations to develop culturally relevant prevention and treatment programs.

In 1992, the Foundation adopted the recommendations made in a staff report to the board, which guided its grantmaking throughout the 1990s. In practical terms, the Foundation's programs during most of the decade were structured around four categories of grantmaking:

1. One category focused on research and policy change, gathering prevalence data and developing policies to reduce the harmful effects of alcohol, drugs, and tobacco. The Bridging the Gap program (1992–2006) supports surveys to track the prevalence of alcohol, drug, and tobacco use among the young, as well as studies of state and local practices aimed at curbing such use. The Substance Abuse Policy Research Program (1994–2007) funds studies on policies or the policy implications of practices aimed at curbing the harmful effects of alcohol, drug, and tobacco use. The program, and its predecessor, the Tobacco Policy Research and Evaluation Program, documented, for example, the effect of increased tobacco taxation on lowering smoking rates.

2. Another category aimed at building the fields of alcohol, drug, and tobacco prevention and treatment. The Foundation funded the creation of the Center on Addiction and Substance Abuse at Columbia University to conduct and disseminate research that focused attention on alcohol and drug addiction, as well as on the means to prevent and treat it (1991–2002). It also funded Join Together to provide technical assistance and a communications strategy to disseminate the latest research and findings to prevention and treatment practitioners (1991–2005). Join Together On Line, created in 1991, was ahead of the curve in using Web-based technology to report on innovation. The Developing Leadership in Reducing Substance Abuse program (1998–2007) was created to train leaders who could advance research on the prevention and treatment of alcohol, drug, and tobacco problems. Innovators Combating Substance Abuse (1998–2006) honored creativity and exemplary accomplishment in understanding, preventing, and treating alcohol, drug, and tobacco issues. Recipients of the Innovators award have advanced alcohol screening in emergency departments, employed art to communicate the consequences of addiction, and led innovations in clean indoor air policies.

3. Yet another category focused on prevention. The Community Anti-Drug Coalitions of America (1996–2005) trained thousands of volunteer members of community coalitions to use the latest research findings on preventing drug and alcohol use among young people. Free to Grow (1992–2005) was created to build on the Head Start program and mobilize parents and community leaders to become aware of and combat the misuse of alcohol and drugs.

4. A final category focused on preventing underage alcohol use. The A Matter of Degree program (1995–2007) mobilizes colleges and neighboring communities to work together to curb drinking on and near campus. The Reducing Underage Drinking Through Coalitions program funds state and community coalitions to reduce drinking among high school students. The Center for Alcohol Marketing to Youth (2002–2006) analyzes target audiences for television, radio, and print advertising sponsored by the alcoholic beverage industry. Its findings documented the presence of alcohol advertising whose target audience represents a disproportionately large share of people under twenty-one.

The programs funded by the Foundation during this second phase were based on the view that alcohol, drug, and tobacco use is deeply rooted in complex individual and societal norms and that this behavior can be changed through societal interventions that seek to decrease access to harmful substances. This view sees addiction as a behavior that has health risks rather than as an illness that is preventable and amenable to treatment. Prevention, therefore, is focused on the behavior and the environment of individuals, as it might be with any other problem that is primarily social in nature. In addressing other chronic medical conditions, the focus of prevention is often on the interaction of biological, genetic, behavioral, and environmental factors. Consistent with the perspective that views addiction as a social problem is the relative absence of emphasis on treatment. Most preventable health conditions are accompanied by well-developed treatment protocols and delivery systems addressing illness that has not been successfully prevented. Emergency departments, for example, are poised to treat accident victims who didn't wear seat belts; insurance pays for medications that mitigate diabetes when nutrition and exercise do not succeed. In the case of drug and alcohol addiction, only episodic attention had been given to the quality or the availability of treatment.

—⟋⟍— Phase III: The Impact Framework— Addiction Prevention and Treatment

In the 1990s, alcohol and drug use essentially stabilized when compared with the rates of the previous two decades. Between 81 and 84 percent of people twelve and older reported using alcohol in this decade, compared with a high of 89 percent in 1979.[9] Drug use, while relatively stable through the 1990s, at between 33 and 36 percent for the lifetime use of any drug, increased slightly from the 31 percent reported in 1979. In 1993, Bill Clinton took office as president, and he publicly acknowledged his family's history of addiction.

Professionals in the field of prevention and treatment welcomed the new administration's support for the idea of reducing the demand for alcohol and drugs among young Americans. The hope was that this support would result in a new policy aimed at reducing demand and also in new resources to combat addiction. These heightened expectations went unmet, however. There were no significant new resources and no significant change in the policy of previous administrations, which allocated two-thirds of every government dollar spent in the so-called War on Drugs to interdicting the supply in foreign lands or on the streets of America. For the most part, the 1990s were socially conservative years, a time when individuals who were dependent on alcohol or drugs were denied disability benefits and addicted pregnant women were, in some states, incarcerated for child endangerment.

Still, the decade did see a significant growth in the scientific understanding of addiction and in the means to prevent and treat it. Both the National Institute on Alcohol Abuse and Alcoholism and the National Institute on Drug Abuse developed research programs that advanced the understanding of the brain's response to alcohol and other specific drugs; research also advanced the understanding of pharmaceuticals that block or neutralize the effects of alcohol and drugs on the brain. The neurological dimension became crucial to understanding addiction as a medical condition. Research established a genetic link to alcohol problems and dependence. Moreover, the National Institute of Drug Abuse and the federal Substance Abuse and Mental Health Services Administration commissioned the Institute of Medicine to conduct a study to determine and recommend how the positive results of clinical trials of pharmaceutical and behavioral interventions could be quickly adopted by treatment organizations. By 1998, the concept of addiction as "a brain disease" began to achieve prominence among professionals in the field.

The challenge was to get what was known to be effective into generally accepted practice. Building on the recommendations of the Institute of Medicine report, *Bridging the Gap Between Practice and Research,* the National Institute on Drug Abuse and the Substance Abuse and Mental Health Services Administration created initiatives designed to translate research into practice. Both linked treatment organizations and professionals directly with clinical researchers in networks created to design, conduct, and disseminate proven interventions. The model was lifted directly from the clinical trial network of the National Cancer Institute.

These developments provided the external political and scientific context that shaped the third phase of the Robert Wood Johnson Foundation's work with alcohol and drug prevention and treatment.

A staff report to the board in 2000 and a new programming framework—drawing directly from the reservoir of scientific understanding of neurology, biology, and the psychosocial dimensions of addiction—described the role that dopamine receptors in the brain play in satisfying reward centers and cravings; the medications and proven clinical interventions available to treat addiction; and the significant gap between need, on the one hand, and available resources (including insurance) on the other. Viewing addiction as a chronic medical condition, the report concluded by recommending that the Foundation give priority to increasing access to quality treatment.

Even before this report, however, the Foundation had begun to move in a new direction with a $21 million five-year program called Reclaiming Futures, which was authorized in 1999. The program aimed at helping adolescents caught up in the criminal justice system because of alcohol or drugs remain with their families and in school. To build connections among courts, families, treatment resources, and schools, the program provides training for judges, probation officers, and counselors as well as technical assistance and financial resources for courts and treatment agencies.

After the 2000 report, the Foundation authorized a series of new programs. Paths to Recovery, authorized in 2001, is a $9.5 million five-year program that, among other things, seeks to redesign admission processes to promote quick access for patients, revamp intake systems to minimize intrusion and redundancy, and deploy counselors to increase retention in treatment programs. In 2002, the federal Substance Abuse and Mental Health Services Administration became a full partner in this effort through an initiative called Strengthening Treatment Access and Retention, effectively doubling the program's size. Today there are more than forty treatment organizations, four states, and three managed care organizations participating in the program. Another Foundation-funded program, the $3 million, four-year Resources for Recovery, which began in 2002, aims at maintaining or increasing the resources available to prevent and treat addiction, even at a time when states face severe fiscal constraints. It provides funds for experts in state financing to help the states draw full potential benefits from the major federal and state programs targeted to addiction prevention and treatment.

Other programs that the Foundation funded in the early 2000s were aimed at developing treatment guidelines for adolescent services; studying the implications of California's Proposition 36 (approved by 61 percent of the voters in 2001, Prop 36 mandated treatment programs rather than jail for people convicted of minor drug offenses); and developing, in conjunction with governmental and nongovernmental partners, initial performance measures of effective treatment that can guide the buyers of drug treatments. Also, in response to a growing number of studies that showed the Drug Abuse Resistance Education program, or DARE, to be ineffective, the Foundation funded a $13 million, five-year effort to redesign the DARE curriculum.

In January 2003, Risa Lavizzo-Mourey, who had recently become the Foundation's president and chief executive officer, presented the board with an "impact framework" to guide the Foundation's grantmaking. Improving the quality of addiction treatment was one of eight strategic objectives set forth in the statement. Specifically, the Foundation sought to improve the quality of addiction treatment by "increasing the number of addiction treatment settings that employ proven interventions."[10] In carrying out the strategy, the Foundation would identify and address barriers to receiving effective care, including organizational obstacles that discourage continued patient engagement and reimbursement practices that discourage the adoption of effective interventions. It would also focus on the need to recognize and act on addiction as a chronic illness.

As one indication of the change in emphasis (and to avoid reinforcing the stigma of addiction), the name of the team working on this new approach within the Foundation was changed from the Alcohol and Illegal Drugs Team to the Addiction Prevention and Treatment Team. Also, the term "substance abuse" was dropped and replaced by such terms as "alcohol or drug problem or addiction" and "substance use disorder." The change in language reinforced the view that addiction is a health condition and avoided the stigmatizing implications of words such as "abuse," and "illicit"—terms better suited to a social problem addressed in the criminal justice system.

In the two years since the board adopted the impact framework, the Foundation has taken a number of steps to reach its objective of increasing the use of proven treatment practices:

First, grants were made to develop program-level measures of such practices. The aim is to work with federal and other partners to have a standard set of indicators for proven practices that can be included in national surveys of treatment programs. To date, the National Quality Forum, an organization in Washington, D.C., that develops standards for measuring health care improvement, has held a workshop that identified five practical candidates for inclusion in surveys:

- The appropriate use of screening and brief intervention tools
- Assessment of patients with alcohol and opiate-specific diagnoses for pharmacologic interventions
- Availability of proven behavioral interventions, such as motivational interviewing and contingency management
- The use of aftercare and follow-up to maintain engagement
- The use of "wraparound" supports such as job training and transitional housing and child care

Second, federal, provider, consumer, and research groups have met and begun to identify principles for a demonstration program that will help treatment programs remove the obstacles to adopting proven practices.

Third, since the states, through health, child welfare, transitional assistance, and criminal justice programs, are the single largest purchasers and regulators of addiction treatment, a set of principles has been identified that can be used in a demonstration initiative to encourage states to use their influence to improve the quality of treatment. Examples of these principles include

- Buying services from networks rather than individual programs so that patients can move seamlessly across levels of care managed by different providers
- Identifying and modifying policies that unintentionally discourage quality—such as reimbursement practices that prohibit payment for medication while reimbursing other services
- Promoting diversity to better serve patients whose language, cultural, racial, or other attributes are different from those of the providers of treatment
- Promoting practices that increase the role of the patients in managing the treatment and aftercare for their condition

Even as phase III programs (those treating addiction as a chronic condition) are being developed, many phase II programs (those viewing addiction as a behavioral and societal issue) are being continued. These include the Partnership for a Drug-Free America, Community Anti-Drug Coalitions of America, the Center on Addiction and Substance Abuse, and Join Together, as well as the programs focused on reducing underage drinking. For programs whose funding is completed, such as Free to Grow, the Foundation is working to consolidate the knowledge gained and to share what was learned. For programs that continue, especially research and field-building initiatives such as the Substance Abuse Policy Research Program and Bridging the Gap, the Foundation is striving to align the remaining work with the phase III objectives.

—ɯ— The Road Ahead

The Foundation's programming in the fields of alcohol and drug addiction will no doubt continue to evolve and reflect external events, current science, and internal perspectives. The Foundation is committed to increasing the number of treatment settings that employ evidence-based interventions. In addition to developing new programs, the Foundation recognizes the importance of maintaining the momentum of the earlier investments in the field.

Over the long run, the Foundation is looking toward an approach to treating drug and alcohol addiction that is based on a widely accepted model of treating chronic illness. This model has five core components:

Community Policies and Resources

These provide the context in which prevention, early intervention, treatment, and aftercare occur. In the past, an eclectic combination of practices developed, based on views of alcohol and drug use that ranged from criminal behavior to willful act to bio-psycho-social condition. Such views have led, in some instances, to policies that dictate the incarceration of drug users and then limit the educational, health, and other benefits needed for successful aftercare. In other instances, prevention efforts are managed exclusively by local law enforcement officials and are unconnected to screening or primary care opportunities. In yet others, policies governing health insurance allow the exclusion or the restriction of benefits and services for persons who seek help for alcohol and drug addiction. The future requires a continuum of prevention, screening, early intervention, treatment, and aftercare, supported by policies that prevent and treat addiction to alcohol or drugs rather than punish the people who are addicted.

A Responsive Delivery System

The delivery system should be available when the patient needs it and offer the level of care required by the patient at the time. Today's addiction prevention and treatment system is an aggregation of some fourteen thousand programs across the country. It lacks the capacity for coordinating care on behalf of a patient. The financially fragile system is still steeped as much in belief systems as in the science of prevention and treatment. Strengthening the system through infrastructure development, consolidation where it is appropriate, adoption of proven approaches, and use of quality improvement practices is critical to bringing about a responsive delivery system.

Clinical Information Systems

These systems provide the ability to consider all dimensions of a patient's needs over time. For alcohol and drug addiction diagnoses, privacy protections have been in place for many years, modeled on the anonymity principles of Alcoholics Anonymous. These provisions have served to protect patients from stigma and discrimination in the workplace and the community, but they have also served to isolate clinical information about addiction from other health-related conditions. Integrating clinical information, within the privacy protections of the law, is important not only to treat addiction effectively but also to treat other medical conditions that are affected by the use of alcohol and drugs.

Decision Supports

Decision supports guide and promote effective practice in any prevention or treatment activity. A sizable literature has shown what practices are effective in preventing and treating alcohol and drug misuse. For example, the Substance Abuse and Mental Health Service Administration's Treatment

Improvement Protocol Series and the National Registry of Effective Programs and Practices document approaches and protocols applicable to preventing and treating alcohol and drug problems. The challenge is adopting what has been shown to work.

Active and Engaged Consumers

Committed patient-participants are essential to monitoring progress, educating others, and advocating for the resources needed to manage chronic illness. On one hand, the addiction treatment field excels at creatively using patients. The self-help movement represents an aftercare peer support network that is the envy of any system that treats chronic illness. Until recently, as many as 50 percent of the counselors working in addiction treatment were themselves at one time problem users or were addicted to alcohol and drugs.[11] On the other hand, alcohol and drug treatment programs are known for rules that forbid patient contact with social and family networks and discharge patients for violating essentially procedural rules or not complying with protocols and similar practices that marginalize the patient. A newly emerging consumer movement has the potential to build on the strengths derived from the heavy involvement that consumers traditionally have had in this field and to become a force for more and better resources at the community level.

—ɯ— Spanning the Prevention-Treatment Divide

Every year, as the new school year begins, the government releases data from tracking surveys that detail past month, past year, and lifetime reported use of alcohol and a large number of specific drugs by age group for people twelve and older. The reports cite variations in reported use from the previous year that, depending on the direction of the trends, are cause for alarm or for cautious celebration and become focal points for further action.[12]

Less often is a long-term view taken on prevalence in these reports. That long-term view would show generational changes in drug and alcohol use but not wide variation of use patterns within ten-year intervals.[13] If there is a relatively constant rate of prevalence for alcohol and drug use over many generations, it would seem logical to conclude that multiple strategies are needed until sufficient knowledge is gained about the interaction of neurological, biological, and genetic predispositions with the social context that results in addiction. The divide between those who view addiction to alcohol and drugs as totally preventable and those who view it as totally treatable has been based more on assertion and belief than on science. Learning from other chronic illness, the nation's health authorities have put in place broad prevention strategies and education aimed at informing the behaviors of Americans to exercise, eat right, and avoid environmental and behavioral risks. These are demonstrated approaches to reducing cardiovascular disease and diabetes. In addition to this knowledge and these demonstrated approaches to preventing illness, the nation maintains a standing capacity for treating these conditions in both primary and specialty care settings. Now the nation needs the same capacity for reducing exposure to alcohol and drugs and for preventing and treating addiction.

Notes

1. Office of Applied Studies. "Highlights of Findings." *2002 National Survey on Drug Use and Health.* Rockville, Md.: Substance Abuse and Mental Health Services Administration (SAMHSA). DHHS Publ. No. SMA 03-3774, 2002, pp. 6–10.

2. McGinnis, J. M., and Foege, W. H. "Mortality and Morbidity Attributable to the Use of Substances in the United States." *Proceedings of the Association of American Physicians,* 1998, *111*(2), 109–118.

3. D'Onofrio, G., et al. "Patients with Alcohol Problems in the Emergency Department, Part 1: Improving Detection." *Academic Emergency Medicine,* 1998, *5*(12), 1200–1209.

4. Walsh, D. C., et al. "A Randomized Trial of Treatment Options for Alcohol-Abusing Workers." *New England Journal of Medicine,* 1991, 325, 775–782.

5. Office of Applied Studies. Table 2.8, Trends in Reporting Alcohol and Tobacco Use in the Past Month by Age Group: 1979–1998. *National Household Survey on Drug Abuse: Main Findings 1998.* Rockville, Md.: Substance Abuse and Mental Health Services Administration (SAMHSA). DHHS Publ. No. SMA 99-3327, 2002, p. 31.

6. NIAAA, Press Release. "Youth Drinking Trends Stabilize, Consumption Remains High." Sept. 14, 2004, p. 1.

7. For a full discussion of the parents' movement, see Massing, M. *The Fix.* New York: Simon and Schuster, 1998, pp. 166–176.

8. Wielawski, I. "The Fighting Back Program." *To Improve Health and Health Care. Vol. VII: The Robert Wood Johnson Foundation Anthology.* San Francisco, Jossey-Bass, 2004.

9. Office of Applied Studies. Table 2.2, Trends in Percentage of Respondents Aged 12 and Older Reporting Drug Use in Their Lifetime: 1979–1998. *National Household Survey on Drug Abuse: Main Findings 1998.* Rockville, Md.: Substance Abuse and Mental Health Services Administration (SAMHSA). DHHS Publ. No. SMA 99-3327, 2002, p. 25.

10. In January, 2005, the Foundation's board of trustees approved extending the time frame of this work through 2009.

11. Roman, P., et al. National Treatment Center Study, Summary Report. University of Georgia (Athens campus), Sept. 2004, p. 8; see also Northwest Frontier Addiction Technology Transfer Center. *Advancing the Current State of Addiction Treatment: A Regional Needs Assessment of Substance Abuse Treatment Professionals in the Pacific Northwest.* Salem, Ore.: Author, 2004, p. 18.

12. Monitoring the Future survey; for a complete description, see (www.monitoring thefuture.org).

13. Office of Applied Studies. Table 2.6, Trends in Percentage Reporting Drug Use in the Past Year, by Age Group: 1979–1998. *National Household Survey on Drug Abuse: Main Findings 1998.* Rockville, Md.: Substance Abuse and Mental Health Services Administration (SAMHSA). DHHS Publ. No. SMA 99-3327, p. 29.

A Closer Look

Students Run LA

Paul Brodeur

Editors' Introduction

Every year, the *Anthology* devotes a chapter to one of the smaller projects that the Foundation funds. These are often innovative projects that take place in a single location and serve people in need. Many are funded through the Local Initiative Funding Partners, a program in which the Robert Wood Johnson Foundation collaborates with local foundations that have identified promising opportunities. Past volumes of the *Anthology* have featured chapters on an alternative high school in Albuquerque for young people with drug and alcohol problems,[1] a San Francisco project that provides care to homeless pregnant women,[2] the efforts of leaders in Gallup, New Mexico, to reduce drinking in that city,[3] and a project in Chicago that takes a public health approach to reducing gun violence.[4]

This volume highlights Students Run LA, a project that gives at-risk Los Angeles students the chance to compete in the City of Los Angeles Marathon. Participating students work toward a common goal—competing in the marathon—and in the process of training for and running the event, they learn self-discipline and feel the sense of accomplishment that comes from reaching a difficult goal. Superficially, the program is about running a race; in a more profound sense, it is about building character. More than 16,000 students have run the Los Angeles Marathon. As the chapter's author, award-winning journalist Paul Brodeur, observes, the graduation rate of those students far exceeds the graduation rate for students in the Los Angeles Unified School District.

The Robert Wood Johnson Foundation was not involved at the beginning of Students Run LA, which, as often happens, resulted from the efforts of caring and charismatic individuals. Through the Local Initiative Funding Partners program, the Foundation was able to play a role in extending the program, which had previously been limited to high schools, to middle schools throughout the city. The staff of the Local Initiative program judged Students Run LA to be so promising that a second grant was awarded to enable the program's directors to develop materials that could be used by other cities that picked up the idea. Philadelphia has already done so with Students Run Philly Style, which received financial support through the Local Initiative Funding Partners program.

---

1. Diehl, D. "Recovery High School." In *Anthology, Vol. V* (2002).
2. Diehl, D. "The Homeless Prenatal Program." In *Anthology, Vol. VII* (2004).
3. Brodeur, P. "Combating Alcohol Abuse in Northwestern New Mexico: Gallup's Fighting Back and Healthy Nations Programs." In *Anthology, Vol. VI* (2003).
4. Diehl, D. "The Chicago Gun Violence Program." In *Anthology, Vol. VIII* (2005).

6

:30 A.M. on Sunday morning, October 17, 2004, in downtown Los Angeles. Some two thousand middle and high school runners from the Los Angeles Unified School District are milling about in Grand Hope Park, which is situated behind the Fashion Institute of Design and Merchandising between Grand Avenue and Hope Street, where two dozen yellow school buses provided by Laidlaw Transit Services have delivered them from all over the metropolitan area and its sprawling suburbs. Almost all of the runners are being drenched by a chilling rain that has swept in overnight from the Pacific, and many are wearing homemade ponchos—trash bags with holes cut out for heads and arms. In spite of the weather, enthusiasm seems undampened. Gossip and laughter are the order of the day as youngsters greet classmates and rush about to find friends and relatives who have come to watch them participate in a five-kilometer (3.1-mile) training race—the second of several monthly runs to be held in preparation for the twentieth annual twenty-six-mile-385-yard 2005 Los Angeles Marathon, which will take place in early March. Many of the young runners have picked up and donned T-shirts with pink and green lettering reading "Students Run LA"—an after-school fitness program for at-risk students that has been in operation for sixteen years. Most of them come from low-income families. Fifty-two percent are boys; 48 percent are girls. Seventy-one percent have Latino backgrounds; 12 percent are Anglo. The remainder are mostly of Asian, African American, Pacific Islander, and Native American descent.

By 8:00 A.M. the rain has stopped, the skies have begun to brighten, and teacher-coaches wearing yellow jerseys, who are also running in the upcoming race, are beginning to round up their charges. Some of the youngsters are performing stretching exercises by leaning one palm and then the other against a wall of the Institute of Design, and pulling up on the instep of the opposite ankle. Others are jogging in place. By 8:30, the runners are massed behind the starting line on Grand Street, stamping their feet and clapping their hands to chanting and music from a sound system, before listening to the national anthem sung in fine style by a large African American lady on a reviewing stand draped in red and blue bunting.

A few moments later, the start signal is given and the runners are off on a course that encompasses some two dozen city blocks. Within fifteen minutes or so, the leaders appear around a corner several hundred yards away, run down a two-block-long homestretch along Grand Street, and cross the finish line. As expected, they are the older and more experienced runners. During the next forty-five minutes, other runners round the corner and stream steadily toward the finish line. Some are striding easily, others are plodding, still others are walking, and a few have stopped moving altogether and are standing in place, heads down, hands on knees as they try to regain their strength—a dilemma not uncommon in the late stages of an early-season training race for which many participants, who have not been running during the summer, are unprepared. But there has been one electrifying moment early in the event as a tiny boy of Asian descent, who can't be more than four and a half feet tall, rounds the corner into the homestretch at a pace that attracts attention. Little legs pumping, elbows keeping time, head up, eyes looking neither right nor left, short black hair standing on end as if energized by current, this kid is *motoring!* He is putting on a finishing sprint such as no other runner has before or after him. In the two-block homestretch, he is passing dozens of runners. Runners half again as tall as he, runners whose legs he could almost pass between, runners who look at him as if they can't believe how fast he's going. Spectators near the finish line have seen him coming and they are shouting and applauding. At the line, he raises his arms and disappears into the crowd. Some minutes later, he can be seen squatting on his heels by a wall of the Institute of Design, head down, elbows on knees as he regains his breath. A man—father or older brother?—kneels beside him, puts an arm around his shoulder, says something into his ear.

The boy nods, raises his head, smiles a smile of triumph.

—〰— A Pioneer

The Los Angeles Marathon celebrated its twentieth anniversary in March 2005, and students from Los Angeles schools have been running in it since 1987. That they have been doing so is to the credit of a man named Harry Shabazian, who has been a social studies teacher at the Boyle

Heights Continuation High School in East Los Angeles for twenty-one years. (Continuation schools have been established throughout California to enable at-risk students who have fallen behind in their credits for one reason or another—usually poor attendance or getting into trouble—to work largely one-on-one with teachers in order to master the basic skills of reading and writing by completing a curriculum of written assignments.) A swarthy, mustachioed, and heavily bearded man of Armenian descent, Shabazian was born in Sofia, Bulgaria, spent part of his early childhood in Beirut, Lebanon, and came to the United States at the age of nine, in 1968, when his family settled in the Hollywood section of Los Angeles. He attended Hollywood High School and California State University, Northridge, where he got his teaching credentials. His position at the Boyle Heights Continuation High School—a pair of stucco-coated concrete bungalows—has been his first and only paid teaching job. The walls of his classroom are covered with photographs of student runners, as well as signs with warnings, such as "Do Drugs? Stay Stupid," and graphic photographs showing birth-deformed babies born to teenage mothers who have become addicted to drugs.

A few days before the five-kilometer training race, Shabazian can be heard handing out tough love to a boy and a girl who have been skipping classes. "I know what you're up to," he tells them, with a scowl. "You think you can beat the system, but let me tell you, all you're going to beat is yourselves. So let's do ourselves a favor, come to class, and get the work done!" He is wearing a blue baseball cap, blue shorts, sandals, and a white T-shirt emblazoned on the back with a shark swimming among baitfish. When he sits down to talk, he is blunt, voluble, and exuberant as he remembers his early days at Boyle Heights.

> I knew this was going to be a rough place from the get-go. It was full of tough kids who'd been kicked out of other high schools. The two teachers before me had quit in frustration. I was only twenty-five, and most of the kids I was trying to teach were seventeen—not all that much of an age difference. Right off the bat, I changed my name to Harry. My real name is Hachick, which means "Little Cross," after my grandfather, who was called Hach, or "Big Cross." But I knew I'd never make it with the kids here if they had to call me Hachick, so I called

myself Harry, after a high school history teacher who'd been a mentor of mine. One reason I was able to bond with the kids was that, like most of them— 95 percent of whom are of Latino origin—I also had to learn English as a second language. Another reason was that I connected early on with a streetwise kid named Richard. In the mornings, I was Richard's teacher; in the afternoons, I was his pupil. Richard clued me in on the gang scene in East LA, and it was largely because of him that I was able to convince the other students I was not some kind of cop.

Shabazian goes on to say that three weeks before the 1986 marathon he and two friends decided on the spur of the moment to enter it and try to finish. "My colleagues and I had trained for the race with only a ten-mile run, so we were ill-prepared," he recalls.

By mile fifteen, the euphoria had worn off and I had begun to develop cramps and aches in body parts I didn't even know I had. At that point, I didn't think I could go on. Sweat was turning into salt on my face, and I felt almost delirious. But word had got out around school that we were going to run the marathon, so a bunch of kids had come out to watch, and when the downed runner bus— that's a vehicle marathon officials send around to pick up runners who can't continue—slowed down behind me, as if to take me on board, I took a look at the discouraged faces of the people inside and somehow got myself up and running again. It took me four hours and forty-five minutes to cross the finish line, but when I did someone handed me a metal celebration coin that looked like a laundry token, and suddenly I felt a wonderful sense of accomplishment. When I came to school the next day, I could barely walk, but my kids were incredibly excited. All they wanted to talk about was the marathon.

Toward the end of that year, one of Shabazian's students asked him if he was going to run the marathon again. "To be truthful, it had been such a painful experience I hadn't thought about it much," he recalls with a grin.

Then it occurred to me that it would be great if I could persuade some of the kids to do it with me. Finally, two girls and five boys signed up for the 1987 marathon. What motivated them was that I was going to do it with them. I was not remotely qualified to be a running coach, of course, and totally uncertain about how we should train, so I read a bunch of running magazines and we wound up running a bunch of preparation races. As things turned out, minors below the age of eighteen were not allowed to run in the marathon, so we had to fudge their ages in the entry papers. We held a car wash to pay for the entry fees and for cheap running shoes that cost about twenty bucks a pair. In the end, six of my seven kids finished the marathon. A girl who had to quit had been so excited at the prospect she'd gone out to celebrate the night before, didn't get home till after midnight, couldn't sleep, and was forced to drop out at mile seven. I stayed with her till the end and then caught up with the others at mile seventeen, where the toughest part of the marathon begins. We went on as a group and finished together. Running as a group is very important. It gives everyone the mental strength to continue. As for the kids who finished that year and in following years, there has been an extraordinary benefit. They have a totally different view about school and what they are expected to accomplish here. Their attendance and grades improve remarkably. They set goals for themselves. They graduate. They go to college. I tell them there are more millionaires in the U.S.A. than people who have finished the marathon. For all I know, that may not be true, but they love to hear it.

Shabazian gives a booming laugh as he remembers this possibly dubious exhortation and the fact that the number of students from Boyle Heights who finished the marathon was six in 1987 and twelve the following year and eighteen in 1989.

I ran fifteen consecutive marathons with kids from my school, and by the time I quit almost all of them were crossing the finish line. Now that I reflect back on those years, I realize that the real transformation in these young people takes place during the months of training, when they are setting the goal of running the marathon and preparing to do it. Nowadays, we're taking students as young as fifth-graders to climb Mount Whitney in the Sierras, which at fifteen thousand feet is the highest in the continental United States. Back in 1995, we took twenty students to meet Sir Edmund Hillary, who was in the U.S. to promote mountain climbing and the preservation of the Himalayas. Everyone wants to be recognized in this life, and it means a lot to these kids, who often come from poverty and broken homes, to know that they can run the marathon, climb tall mountains, meet icons such as Hillary, and be watched, talked about, and written about.

Shabazian falls silent a moment before continuing. "Of course, one shouldn't take things too seriously," he says. "I'll be running the 2005 marathon with some former students. We plan to stop off at a McDonald's in the middle of the race so we can have a breather and a sugar rush from apple pie, French fries, and a soda."

—ɯ— The Development of Students Run LA

If Shabazian deserves credit for the brainstorm that led to Students Run LA, two other teachers—Paul Trapani and Eric Spears—should be credited with demonstrating how to raise money and obtain media coverage for a student running program that could be spread to other schools. At the time, Trapani and Spears were working at the Aliso Continuation High School (which was renamed John R. Wooden High School in 2005) in the San Fernando Valley. When the two men read about what Shabazian and his students had done in a school district newsletter, they decided to follow suit, and in 1989 they ran the marathon with some of their students. Since then, they have run many more Los Angeles marathons with their charges—Trapani has run seven and Spears has run seventeen—and today both of them are co-ordinators of the Students Run LA program, with the task of providing guidance and assistance to the 250 teacher-leaders who coach runners in more than 150 schools that now participate in the program. They are helped in this endeavor by Jim Fiorenza, a volunteer transportation co-ordinator, who makes sure that during each month of the training season more than two thousand student runners will be transported on time to the scheduled events. In addition, they are assisted by an administrative staff led by Marsha Charney, executive director of Students Run LA, Rosny Mandell, assistant director, Nikki Carelli, program director, and Ginny Gibbs, development director. These women manage the day-to-day details of the program, secure funding and resources, set policy, and provide support to the individual leaders, such as making sure that running shoes, shorts, and T-shirts are available to be picked up by teacher-leaders so they can be delivered on time to student runners in the vast Los Angeles metropolitan area.

Paul Trapani is a husky, handsome man in his early forties who has an easy smile and an affable manner. He earned his teaching degree at California State University, Northridge, and has been a social studies teacher at the Aliso Continuation High School since 1986. "When I heard about what Harry Shabazian had done with his kids, I knew it was something we should be doing here," he said a few days after the ten-kilometer training run.

> I got my colleague Eric Spears involved, and over time we managed to erect a structure around Harry's initial accomplishment by persuading officials of the school district, the marathon, and a wide variety of foundations, businesses, and organizations to give us their support. During our first year, a $2 thousand grant (the first of two such grants) from an auto insurer, Safeco, paid for weekend race fees so our students could join other members of the running community who were training for the 1988 marathon. The following year, a $35 thousand grant from the Milken Family Foundation paid for running shoes, shorts, T-shirts, transportation, and other expenses for the overall program. The kids had already got into the act by contacting various television stations. As a result, Channel 2 covered a pre-race carb dinner prepared by my mother, and then followed a tiny Latina girl named Sylvia as she ran the 1989 marathon the following day.

Trapani went on to say that as the Students Run LA program expanded during the 1990s, an ever-increasing amount of time had to be reserved for making up rosters. He recalled:

> Fortunately, we were able to find someone who showed us how to integrate the rosters and other aspects of the program online. For that reason, we are now able to devote more effort to the all-important business of training and mentoring our student runners, and encouraging them to set and carry out short- and long-term goals. What we celebrate most in this program is perseverance. Some of our kids finish the marathon in four to five hours. Others may take six to seven hours. Still others may require eight hours or more to struggle past the finish line. But almost all of them finish. Imagine being that determined!

Eric Spears is a slender, soft-spoken, and bearded man, who wears his long hair in a ponytail. He remembers that when Paul Trapani and he decided to try to emulate what Harry Shabazian had accomplished, they went to get the advice of an expert in kinesiology (the study of muscles) at California State University, Northridge, who advised against it, saying he didn't think it was healthy for youngsters to run the marathon. However, Spears and Trapani decided that by training with shorter runs they could get the kids in shape, and they finally won the kinesiologist over to their point of view to the extent that he began helping them set weekly mileage goals. "We trained after school, twenty to twenty-five miles a week, and on weekends we ran on trails and bike paths in the San Fernando Valley," Spears recalls. "There were only seven of us the first year, then sixty, and after that the whole program took off."

Spears became principal of the Temescal Canyon Continuation High School in Pacific Palisades in 1994, and since 2000 he has been the principal of the Community Day School Program, which has twenty-nine sites in Greater Los Angeles that require him to do a great deal of freeway driving each day. In spite of his rigorous schedule, he remains deeply committed to and involved in Students Run LA.

> I think most teachers feel a deep sense of joy when they realize that the running program is helping to change young lives. The kids who finish the marathon are no longer languishing. Discipline issues disappear. Attendance and grades improve. The main thing about the program, however, is that it's not really about running. It's about setting goals—short-term goals such as running the marathon, and long-term goals such as attending college—and developing the sense of pride and accomplishment that comes with setting and achieving goals. The program affords youngsters the experience of joining together and the opportunity of building character. Believe me, it is very empowering for the kids who participate in it.

A year after Trapani, Spears, and their students ran their first marathon, Roberta Weintraub, a former president of the Los Angeles Unified School District's Board of Education, as well as a three-time elected member of the board, became interested in the fledgling movement. Thanks largely to her efforts, officials of the Los Angeles Marathon waived their previous prohibition preventing students under the age of eighteen from running in the marathon, as well as the entry fee for Students Run LA runners. In addition, Weintraub persuaded the board to designate Students Run LA as an approved program, and was thus instrumental in spreading it districtwide. Since then, enrollment in and support for the program has increased by leaps and bounds. More than 250 student runners entered the marathon in 1990, and 235 finished it; 450 entered in 1991, and 426 finished; 651 entered in 1992, and 625 finished; and 1,026 entered in 1993, and 996 finished. During that year, Students Run LA became a 501(c)(3) nonprofit organization. Meanwhile, Laidlaw Transit Services made an extraordinary and continuing in-kind donation of all the school buses needed for the program.

By 2004, membership in Students Run LA had doubled, with more than two thousand students starting the marathon and 98 percent of them finishing it. Ninety-seven percent of the seniors who completed the marathon that year graduated, and 90 percent of those went on to attend college and other postsecondary educational institutions. Since Students Run LA was started in 1989, more than 16,000 student runners have completed the Los Angeles Marathon. The average graduation rate is more than 90 percent, as compared with a 65 percent graduation rate for students in the Los Angeles Unified School District.

During the sixteen years since Students Run LA came into being, donations and grants have poured in from various private foundations, corporations, and other organizations to foot the bill for the monthly races that student runners participate in as part of their six-month training regimen. (In addition to a one-mile preliminary race in September and the five-kilometer race in October, the training program includes a ten-kilometer [6.2-mile] run, a fifteen-kilometer [9.3-mile] run, two half-marathons, and a grueling thirty-kilometer [eighteen-mile] race that is held in early February at Hansen Dam in Lake View Terrace, north of the city. Foundation and corporate grants are also used to finance a scholarship and minigrant program. Through this program, Students Run LA provides $500 scholarships to graduating seniors who have completed the marathon, maintained at least a 2.5 grade point average, and demonstrated financial need. The scholarships help students who attend college to pay for books, tuition, and other expenses. The minigrants are awards of up to $300 given to youngsters in grades six through eleven who have completed the marathon and demonstrated financial need. They are used to pay for SAT preparation courses, art classes, math or science programs, and other educational activities. Still other foundation and corporate grants are used to finance special events, such as an annual Girls Day, which has increased female participation in Students Run LA from 37 percent to 48 percent during the past seven years, and an annual leader training conference, which enables the program's volunteer teacher-leaders to meet one another and share experiences and information. Among the major sponsors of these and other Students Run LA activities are the American Honda Motor Company, the California Wellness Foundation, the Los Angeles Police Department, the *Los Angeles Times,* the Los Angeles Unified School District, the California Endowment, the Amateur Athletic Foundation, the Ahmanson Foundation, the Weingart Foundation, the S. Mark Taper Foundation, and the W.M. Keck Foundation.

—w— The Initial Role of the Robert Wood Johnson Foundation

In 1987, thanks largely to the vision and tenacity of Terrance Keenan, then a vice president at the Robert Wood Johnson Foundation, the Foundation created the Local Initiative Funding Partners program, or LIFP, to encourage partnerships with smaller foundations that, like the Robert Wood Johnson Foundation, fund projects in the area of health and health care. Local Initiative Funding Partners is a program of matching grants designed to support collaborative relationships between the Robert Wood Johnson Foundation and local grantmakers that finance innovative community-based projects that serve people who are underserved and at risk. The philosophy guiding the program is the belief that local grantmakers interested in addressing local health care problems have a knowledge of their communities that no national foundation can match.[1]

Between 1988 and the end of 2004, the Robert Wood Johnson Foundation has collaborated through its Local Initiative Funding Partners Program with more than 1,200 local grantmakers to fund 250 projects in all fifty states. During this period, the Foundation has awarded $86 million in LIFP grants that have been matched by funds from local granting coalitions, such as community foundations, family foundations, corporate grantmakers, and others. Local Initiative Funding Partners grants of between $100,000 and $500,000 per project are paid out over a three- to four-year period, and are awarded through a competitive process that begins when a local grantmaker prepares a letter of nomination recommending a local applicant's project, and when the local applicant submits a brief proposal describing the project, together with a one-page preliminary budget. Selected applicants are then invited to submit full proposals, which are reviewed by members of an advisory committee and by the LIFP's program staff. After this review, projects still under consideration receive site visits. By the time of a site visit, there must be clear evidence that matching funds will be in place for the first year, and that local funding sources for subsequent years have been identified.

In September 1997, Gary Yates, president and chief executive officer of the California Wellness Foundation—a longtime supporter of Students Run LA—wrote to Pauline M. Seitz, a former senior program officer at the Robert Wood Johnson Foundation, who had become director of the Foundation's Local Initiative Funding Partners program, nominating Students Run LA for funding through the Local Initiative program. "We believe that Students Run LA represents an innovative and effective approach to promoting health and preventing substance abuse among youth, including low-income, special needs, and high-risk students," Yates told Seitz. Some idea of the need for such an approach can be seen in the narrative section of a proposal entitled "Students Run LA Middle School Campaign," which Students Run LA's Marsha Charney sent to Seitz on December 10, 1997. Citing a report called *Children's ScoreCard Los Angeles County 1996,* Charney wrote that 28 percent of the 2,577,819 children in Los Angeles County lived below the poverty level. Citing statistics furnished by the Los Angeles Police Department, she went on to point out that as of January 1996, there were 58,659 gang members in Los Angeles County, whose primary activity involved the use and sale of drugs. According to the Los Angeles Police Department, the average age of a gang member was sixteen; most had joined a gang by the age of twelve; 90 percent had been arrested at least once by the age of eighteen; 95 percent did not finish high school; and 60 percent were either dead or in prison by the age of twenty.

After considering the Students Run LA application for funding, the Robert Wood Johnson Foundation, through the Local Initiative program, made a grant of $235,000 in July 1998 for a three-year program that would increase the ranks of student runners to include middle school students between the ages of twelve and fifteen. At the time, the Foundation had not yet embarked on grantmaking to address obesity and physical fitness (in which it has since developed a strong interest), so the program was based on the expectation that training for and running in the marathon would encourage middle school students to build self-esteem, improve nutrition, and avoid the use of tobacco, alcohol, and illegal drugs. In addition to the California Wellness Foundation, local funding partners in the project included the California Community Foundation, the Milken Family Foundation, the Crail-Johnson Foundation, the Bank of America Foundation, the Ralph M. Parsons Foundation, and the Los Angeles Junior Chamber of Commerce.

The initial involvement of the Robert Wood Johnson Foundation with Students Run LA proved to be a great success. During the project, which ran from the beginning of August 1998 until the end of July 2001, more than 1,000 middle school students were enrolled in Students Run LA's marathon-running program. "All we had to do was put the word out," Martha Charney recalls. "The middle schools were already knocking on our door. What we had to be careful about was not to push the younger students too hard or too far. In many instances, therefore, we allowed them to set the half-marathon as their goal during their first year in the program, and to continue in the full-marathon project during the following year."

—ᴠᴠ— Replicating Students Run LA

In June 2002, Pauline Seitz telephoned Marsha Charney to get her thoughts on the possibility of nationwide replication. Charney told Seitz that she felt Students Run LA did not have the organizational infrastructure needed for national replication, but that she and her colleagues would be interested in exploring a special opportunities grant to describe the program experience, evaluate the results to date, and describe the lessons learned in going from a $35-thousand-a-year project to a $1-million-a-year nonprofit. Seitz and Charney then discussed the need for a Students Run LA "toolkit"— a package of instructional materials that local communities interested in starting similar marathon-running programs could adapt.

In January 2003, Charney sent Seitz a six-page proposal entitled "Replication of the Students Run LA Program," in which she listed ten "ingredients" that she and her colleagues had identified as necessary to operate and sustain a student marathon-running project. She described the first two as "essential, critical, irreplaceable, and non-negotiable." The ten ingredients can be summarized as follows:

- One or a few enthusiastic, energetic, and passionate teacher-leaders who are committed to helping at-risk young people become strong, resilient, motivated students, and who are interested in training for and running in a marathon themselves.

- Students aged twelve to nineteen who are willing to try out the concept.

- School principals who will support the use of school facilities for the teacher-leaders and students to train before and/or after school, and who understand and support the essential goal of the program, which is to teach at-risk youth how to set a goal and achieve it through participation in and completion of a marathon.

- A member or members of the board of education who will not only understand and be advocates for the running program but also provide the imprimatur and resources of the board, which may include funding, insurance, access to transportation, and acceptance as a bona fide activity.

- The leader of the local city marathon, who will accept and support the program, and who will be willing to waive any age or time requirements of that particular marathon.

- A board of directors to help the new organization gain access to the community and acquire resources. Board members should include those with access to government, philanthropies, corporations, health care agencies, and other community agencies and resources.

- A director to administer the program, oversee the staff and budget, develop informational materials, and send out proposals to raise money for the program.

- Sponsors to provide funds and/or products to outfit the initial group of students, who will need good-quality running shoes to train properly.

- Local community races that teacher-leaders and student runners can enter during their training period.

- Local political supporters to help the organization put on its own races (with permits, access, police assistance) and to help with resources at all levels of government.

In her proposal to Seitz, Charney went on to describe a toolkit that would include information on the "who, what, when, where, and why" of creating a student marathon-running program, including descriptions of the Students Run LA philosophy, program structure, seasonal time frame, program costs, strategies for implementation, insurance and liability issues, adult and student responsibilities, evaluation criteria, training for adult leaders, staffing needs, and other essential information. Among the chief components of the package would be a teacher-leader manual explaining how to start a student running group, and what training techniques and schedule to employ; a video describing the experiences and observations of student runners and their teacher-leaders; and a runner's journal and training log that students could use each year while they participate in the program.

In July 2003, the Robert Wood Johnson Foundation awarded a $250,000 grant to Students Run LA for a two-year project during which it would develop an instructional package that would be used to teach other communities how to organize and replicate the Students Run LA program. Development of the toolkit began on August 1, 2003, under the direction of Kristine S. Breese, Student Run LA's project director, who proceeded to review the organization's written materials, hire graphics design personnel, and consult with teacher-leaders to evaluate, modify, and improve a prototype kit. A final model of the toolkit was produced in November 2004, and during 2005 a business plan was developed to determine the essential market for it and the best way to disseminate it. Meanwhile, Students Run LA officials had received inquiries about the toolkit from more than half a dozen cities interested in acquiring it.

The major component of the kit is a brightly colored notebook entitled "Up and Running," which contains well over a hundred pages of instruction on how to start up a marathon-running program, how to train, and how to build confidence, endurance, and self-esteem. The notebook also provides a marathon leaders' handbook that advises teacher-leaders on how to motivate and train young runners. In addition to the notebook, the toolkit contains a video that features Trapani, Spears, Charney, and a number of students talking about the value and success of Students Run LA, as well as a 124-page runner's journal that lists training, nutritional, and safety tips for young runners.

—ᗰ— Students Run Philly Style

In February 2003, Susan Sherman, president and chief executive officer of the Independence Foundation of Philadelphia, visited Students Run LA while attending an annual Grantmakers in Health meeting that was being held in Los Angeles. Impressed by the achievements of the program, she recommended it for consideration by the National Nursing Centers Consortium of Philadelphia—a nonprofit organization with 140 nurse-managed health centers serving two million patients across the United States, including twelve centers located in Philadelphia. Nursing Consortium officials were enthusiastic about the prospect of replicating Students Run LA in Philadelphia, and on November 4, 2003, Sherman wrote Pauline Seitz a letter nominating the organization as a candidate for funding by the Robert Wood Johnson Foundation's Local Initiative Funding Partners program, and committing the Independence Foundation to providing $50,000 a year if the project were approved.

In an executive summary describing the project, which was to be called Students Run Philly Style, Nursing Consortium officials proposed a three-year funding period to create opportunities for up to 400 middle and high school students to participate in a running program that would "improve their health knowledge and behaviors, self-esteem, attitudes about school, and school attendance." In the project narrative, the Consortium officials wrote that 67 percent of the target area's children were African American, 16 percent were Latino, and 15 percent white; that 45 percent of them lived below the federal poverty level; and that 60 percent—18,300 children in all—were at risk of obesity. They also noted that between 2001 and 2002, only 54 percent of Philadelphia students graduated on time (in four years), that more than one in five Philadelphia ninth-graders dropped out of school each year, and that the daily absence rate for high school students was nearly 22 percent.

According to the proposal, the project would initially be implemented in collaboration with two Nursing Consortium centers—the Falls Family Practice and Counseling Network and the Temple Health Connection—which provide vital community health care to low-income, predominately minority populations of eight public housing developments. The two health centers would, in turn, be supported by a variety of organizations—among them the Temple University Partnership Schools, the School District of Philadelphia, the City of Philadelphia Department of Public Health, the Philadelphia Health Management Corporation, the Delaware County Road Runners Club, Students Run LA, and several middle and high schools in North Philadelphia, perhaps the poorest area in the city. During the initial stages of Students Run Philly Style, team leaders would be recruited from neighborhood schools, health centers, and running clubs, and the program would be confined to North Philadelphia. The initial plans called for the program to be expanded to West Philadelphia in the second and third years. However, when a health collaborative in Haddington called To Our Children's Future with Health became a partner, West Philadelphia was included as well. In addition to the Independence Foundation, the local funding partners included the William Penn Foundation, the Philadelphia Foundation, the Philadelphia Health Management Corporation, the Campbell-Oxholm Foundation, the Samuel S. Fels Fund, the Beck Institute for Cognitive Therapy and Research, and the Keystone Mercy Health Plan.

In July 2004, the Robert Wood Johnson Foundation, through the Local Initiative Funding Partners program, awarded a four-year, $495,000 grant to the National Nursing Centers Consortium to undertake the first full-scale replication of the Students Run LA program. However, instead of being a completely school-based program like Students Run LA, Students Run Philly Style has drawn its student runners and adult leaders from a variety of sources—among them support groups for youth, health centers, churches, and after-school programs, as well as several schools. This approach is largely due to the fact that the Philadelphia Marathon is run in November, which means that students who wish to compete in it must train from March to November, including several months during the summer when schools are closed for vacation. Among the races they have entered during their training period are the ten-mile Blue Cross Broad Street Run, held in May, and the 13.1-mile Jefferson Hospital Philadelphia Distance Run, which takes place in September.

During the winter of 2005, Heather McDanel, a long-distance runner who is project director of Students Run Philly Style, and some colleagues undertook to organize the program in earnest, and on Saturday, March 12, seventy-five young runners and thirty-five leaders, who were joined by Eric Spears, Paul Trapani, four-time Olympic middle distance runner Joetta Clark-Diggs, and Pedro Larios, a member of Students Run LA, met for a kickoff celebration that included a twenty-minute Run for Fun along Kelly Drive, along the Schuylkill River. Since then, thirty adult mentors—among them an advocate for the homeless, a Germantown pastor, a Trinidadian soccer player, a school police officer, several running enthusiasts, and some college students—have been paired with groups of eight to ten teenagers with whom they practice at least three times a week, before embarking upon a long run each weekend. Students Run Philly Style is open to students aged twelve to eighteen. Those fifteen and older are trained to run in the marathon, while younger students are trained to run the event as part of four-member relay teams or in the eight-kilometer run associated with the marathon.

~~~ The 2005 Los Angeles Marathon

Meanwhile, the twentieth annual running of the Los Angeles Marathon was held on Sunday, March 6, under clear skies and relatively cool temperatures. More than 25,000 runners competed, of whom 2,250 were members of Students Run LA, including some 700 middle school students whose entry into the marathon had been facilitated by the 1998 grant from the Robert Wood Johnson Foundation's Local Initiative program. A few days before the race, eight of these young runners—all between the ages of eleven and thirteen, and all from Latino backgrounds—gathered in the classroom of thirty-two-year-old Tommy Munoz, their coach and mentor, who has been a sixth-grade history teacher at the Hollenbeck Middle School for five years, and who would be entering the 2005 marathon with fourteen Hollenbeck students. (Hollenbeck, in East Los Angeles, is in the same complex of schools that houses Roosevelt Senior High School and the Boyle Heights Continuation High School.) The eight students— Jessica, Juan, Mireya, Jennifer, Elizabeth, Madeline, Oscar, and Marlene— had trained in arduous conditions; several of the races were run in the cold rain or drizzle that had characterized much of California's winter weather. Most of them agreed, however, that the most difficult race of all was the half marathon that had been held at Newport in December, after a scheduled race at Malibu had been cancelled for lack of permits.

"It poured rain the whole way," Jessica said. "My body was numb."

"My knuckles were white," Oscar said.

"Mine were purple," Jennifer chimed in.

Madeline nodded in agreement. "My hands were swollen."

Elizabeth, a veteran thirteen-year-old runner who had already entered and finished two marathons, smiled a shy smile. "I'm hoping to better my time this year," she announced.

On marathon morning, the 2,250 runners participating in Students Run LA gathered in subterranean ballrooms of the Wilshire Grand Hotel in downtown Los Angeles, where they were issued bright pink caps, T-shirts, and numbered placards. By 7:45 A.M. they had massed behind the starting line at Figueroa and Sixth Street, and after the wheelchair contestants and a select group of top women runners had been allowed to start early, the main race began shortly after 8:00 A.M. preceded by the sound of klaxon horns and the roar of motorcycles ridden by white-helmeted cops of the Los Angeles Police Department. Since slower runners were positioned at the back of the pack, few pink hats were seen during the first fifteen minutes, but by 8:20 they were everywhere in the stream of runners flowing twenty abreast along the four lanes of Figueroa.

The day heated up as the sun rose higher in the sky, and by noontime, when the first student runners began crossing the finish line, the temperature had climbed into the seventies. To afford relief, a fire truck was hosing down tired runners, who were wearing orange ribbons and medals around their necks to signify that they had finished the marathon. Some of the adult runners were limping, some were holding their backs, and a few were being taken away in wheelchairs. As for the Students Run LA members, there were many more smiles than grimaces, many high fives, and much photographing and hugging by proud parents, family members, and friends. In the end, all fourteen of the Hollenbeck Middle School kids who entered the marathon finished, and fully 99 percent of the 2,250 Students Run LA members who entered also finished. Down in the ballroom of the Wilshire Grand, where hundreds of young finishers were stoking up on a post-race lunch of pasta and macaroni, there was a deafening roar of celebratory chatter.

Elizabeth was ecstatic. She had run the marathon in six hours and five minutes—her best time ever.

—ᴡᴡ— Conclusion

The Robert Wood Johnson Foundation made a significant contribution to an already successful program when it financed the entry of middle school students into the Los Angeles Marathon between 1998 and 2001. Since then, the Foundation has undertaken to encourage student marathon running at other locations by funding the writing of a toolkit designed to demonstrate how Los Angeles developed its program, and by financing a full-scale replication of the Students Run LA program in Philadelphia. One of the main ingredients of the success of Students Run LA is that it is school-based, with teacher-leaders who spend time each day with their charges, and who know them on an intimate basis. The question is whether Students Run Philly Style can match the success of the Los Angeles school-based program by drawing upon adult leaders, who may not be as closely connected on a daily basis with young runners as their counterparts on the West Coast. Only time will tell.

Note

1. For a fuller description, see Wielawski, I. M. "The Local Initiative Funding Partners Program." *To Improve Health and Health Care 2000: The Robert Wood Johnson Foundation Anthology.* San Francisco: Jossey-Bass, 1999.

Profile

8

Terrance Keenan: An Appreciation

Digby Diehl

Editors' Introduction

In our efforts to keep the *Anthology* objective and unbiased, we have always had a policy that authors not promote the Robert Wood Johnson Foundation or those who work for it. This chapter represents a departure from that policy. It is an unabashed tribute to the Foundation's most revered staff member. Terry Keenan joined the Robert Wood Johnson Foundation as one of its first employees, and for more than thirty years he has set the standard for creativity, caring, and vision.

Digby Diehl, a noted author and frequent contributor to the *Anthology* series, intertwines the story of Keenan's life with his philosophy of grantmaking and a description of the programs he developed and nurtured. As Diehl observes, Keenan has had an enormous influence on philanthropy both at the Robert Wood Johnson Foundation and nationally.

Although the chapter is focused on Keenan, there is much to be learned from it about the craft of grantmaking. Keenan embodies a human approach to philanthropy. He understands the importance of policy change—and, indeed, his grants contributed to significant policy change in a number of fields—but his insistence on keeping people at the center of grantmaking is what makes him unique. His approach to philanthropy—that the core of foundations' work is helping people in need—is what, in the end, has made Keenan such a beloved and influential figure in the field.

—ᴡ— If you visit Terry Keenan at his modest home in the small village of Newtown, Pennsylvania, you are struck by how much the man lives up to his legend. Throughout the world of philanthropy, and particularly in the realm of health care philanthropy, Keenan is respected as a pioneer of modern grantmaking and a model program officer. He is a man who helped change both the reality and perception of foundations by greatly influencing the development of contemporary grantmaking and foundation policy. As one of the original members of the Robert Wood Johnson Foundation staff in 1972, he played an important role in the institution for more than thirty years.

What is less known about Keenan is that he was the unlikely Indiana Jones of the Robert Wood Johnson Foundation. Keenan fearlessly ventured single-handed into urban jungles and traveled to remote rural outposts to bring health care to communities that were deeply in need. Like the movie character, he used his sharp intellect and academic training to analyze problems and find solutions. With no need of a whip or a gun, Keenan made his shy smile and friendly handshake the face of a giant foundation in small towns and struggling inner-city health projects throughout the country. He is revered as the man who took philanthropy out of the wood-paneled boardrooms and into the narrow alleys, the dirt roads, and the backwaters of America, where the most vulnerable populations needed help.

Keenan, who officially retired in December 2003, continues to be an influence at the Foundation as a special program consultant. At his home, he wears the same tan windbreaker for which he was well-known at the Foundation, with the slight modification of a plaid flannel shirt instead of a white shirt and tie. Keenan is slight of build, perhaps five feet two inches tall. Wisps of white hair grace his otherwise bald head. He wears rimless glasses tinted yellow. Even behind the tinted lenses, his eyes flash with energy and enthusiasm as he speaks, and throughout the conversation he maintains the sort of eye contact and intensity that make you feel that his mission is to persuade you personally. He is no orator, but his manner expresses integrity and thoughtfulness. He repeats many of his noted precepts of grantmaking with an enthusiasm that is fresh and contagious.

If there is a single key to Keenan's extraordinary career in philanthropy, it is a booklet he wrote in 1992, *The Promise at Hand*.[1] This booklet is based on a series of lectures he gave at the Foundation in 1990–1991 as part of its twentieth-anniversary celebration. As Steven Schroeder, who was then the president and chief executive officer of the Foundation, wrote in his introduction, *The Promise at Hand* is "a distillation of the insights developed in [Keenan's] long and fruitful career."

What Makes a Foundation Great?

1. A great foundation is informed and animated by moral purpose.

2. A great foundation accepts responsibility and stewardship for pursuing these purposes.

3. A great foundation walks humbly with its grantees—it acknowledges that their success is the instrument of its own success.

4. A great foundation is deliberate. It is guided by judgment. It acts where there is a need to act. It takes necessary risks—and proceeds in the face of great odds.

5. A great foundation is a resource for both discovery and change. It invests not only in the identification of answers, but also in the pursuit of solutions.

6. A great foundation is accountable. It functions as a public trust—and places its learning and experience in the public domain.

7. A great foundation builds investment partnerships around its goals, creating coalitions of funders—public and private—to multiply its impact.

8. Conversely, a great foundation participates in funding coalitions being organized by other parties to lend its support to purposes requiring multiple funders.

> 9. Finally, a great foundation is self-renewing. It adheres to a constant process of self-reflection and self-assessment. It knows when it needs to change and to adopt measures to improve its performance.
>
> —Terrance Keenan, *The Promise at Hand*

Because Keenan is, in Schroeder's words, "a living embodiment of the best aspects of the Robert Wood Johnson Foundation," his precepts for active philanthropy and foundation ethics in the booklet also reflect his personal standards.

—ᴡᴡ— Early Life

Keenan's diversified early career prepared him surprisingly well for grant-making. He grew up in the bustling artistic community of New Hope, Pennsylvania, the son of Peter Keenan, a Modernist artist of the New Hope School, and a mother who ran the local tearoom. "My father had studied at the Slade School of Fine Art in London, and to support his serious painting—and his five children—he became a sports illustrator for the *Philadelphia Bulletin*," Keenan recalls. "He loved the surroundings of New Hope and the company of the other artists there. The American Impressionist painter John Fulton Folinsbee was one of our neighbors."

He began to follow in his father's artistic footsteps at age ten, when he was selected to exhibit his artwork at a local showing. World War II exposed him to the wider world; he spent the years 1944 to 1946 as a naval aviator, flying as a navigator throughout the South Pacific. When he returned to civilian life, he enrolled at Yale to study English literature. "Yale accepted almost three times as many students as usual in my class [of 1950] because of all the veterans," Keenan notes. "We were doubled up in rooms and the classes were crowded, but I loved the rich learning experiences." He graduated with Phi Beta Kappa honors and pursued each of his interests with such eclecticism that he qualified to teach English, Spanish, French, history, and art appreciation at the Thomas Jefferson prep school in St. Louis, Missouri, for the next five years. He even found time in his youth to become a Golden Gloves boxing contender. Laughing, Keenan insists modestly, "I wouldn't make too much of that. In my weight class, at 145 pounds, you just had to be fast and light on your feet and strong. You really didn't hurt anyone, and no one ever hurt me too badly."

When Keenan moved to New York, in 1955, he worked for the investment firm Merrill Lynch, Pierce, Fenner & Beane, where he was charged with writing the biography of the company's founder, Charles E. Merrill. A year later, exactly ten years after separating from the Navy, he began his long career in philanthropy as a writer for the Ford Foundation, directing the foundation's Office of Reports, under J. Quigg Newton. He joined the Ford Foundation the year it made a groundbreaking blanket distribution of $660 million to all colleges, universities, hospitals, and medical schools in the United States. As Paul Jellinek, a friend and former vice president at the Robert Wood Johnson Foundation, once joked, "For those of you who wonder where Terry got the idea of thinking about scale and thinking big, it started with $660 million from the Ford Foundation."[2] Among his many contributions at Ford, he was chief staff assistant to a trustees committee that wrote a visionary program for the expansion of the foundation in the 1960s.

—〰— Health Care Philanthropy

Health care philanthropy first beckoned to Keenan in May 1965, when he became senior executive associate and board secretary of the Commonwealth Fund. As assistant to Quigg Newton, who had became the fund's president, he was involved with every phase of Commonwealth's activities. "Terry was Quigg's right-hand man, his scribe at the meetings and writer of everything for the foundation from the press releases to the annual reports," says Margaret Mahoney, a longtime friend and colleague of Keenan's. Mahoney is a former vice president of the Robert Wood Johnson Foundation, where she worked with Keenan, president emeritus of the Commonwealth Fund, and currently president of MEM Associates. "When we met, I had an executive associate position at the Carnegie Corporation similar to Terry's, and we became friends almost immediately," she recalls. "I was impressed that his grasp of the big health care issues was deepened by a genuine compassion for the recipients of health care. I think of him as a combination of the sharp-minded Jesuit and the caring parish priest."

What brought Mahoney from the Carnegie and Keenan from Commonwealth together was a conference at the Massachusetts Institute of Technology in the late 1960s on the problems of medical care for the indigent. "The Carnegie Corporation gave the president of MIT $15 thousand to convene a conference on health care for the poor," Mahoney recalls. "Frankly, MIT did not have much interest in medical care or medicine at the time. All of the university medical centers were ignoring this huge problem, and our cities were burning. The report from that meeting more or less confirmed what we already knew. But it brought Carnegie and Commonwealth together to work on the problem. That's how I met Terry."

Frank Karel, former Robert Wood Johnson Foundation vice president for communications, recalls meeting Keenan for the first time in 1965, when he was head of public relations for Johns Hopkins Medical Institutions. "One day, the dean of the medical school, Tommy Turner, called to say that he had to meet with Quigg Newton from the Commonwealth Fund about a grant proposal, and Quigg was bringing some new staff member," Karel says. "The dean wanted me to get this new guy out of the room so that he could be alone with Quigg. That day, I took Terry on the $50 tour of Johns Hopkins, which was a huge sprawling place that covered about five city blocks. We went from the top of every building down into the tunnels below, and Terry loved it. He never stopped asking questions. Terry and I became friends, and the dean got his grant." Two years later, Karel joined Keenan at the Commonwealth Fund as a program officer, and he recalls that they were both struck by how completely independent, arrogant, and disorganized foundations were at that time. "The foundation world was really in disarray," Karel recalls. "They weren't organized; they didn't work together. Terry and I talked about the need for greater responsibility, accountability. This later led Terry to support the evaluation ethic that was championed at the Robert Wood Johnson Foundation from its earliest days. Of course, just a few years after we discussed the problem, Congress took an even dimmer view of foundations in the Tax Reform Act of 1969."

In addition to his concern for the structure and administration of foundations, Keenan began to focus on programmatic areas that would be lifelong pursuits. At the Commonwealth Fund, he had worked on a Clinical Scholars program and academic community health plans and had directed the Commonwealth Fund–Harvard University Press Book Program. "Frank Karel and I were both recruited to work for Commonwealth and began work on the same day in 1968," recalls Annie Lea Shuster, who began as Keenan's assistant at Commonwealth and later became a program officer at the Robert Wood Johnson Foundation. "Much of the thinking for the early Robert Wood Johnson programs was done at Commonwealth. In fact, the three of us would sit around having lunch in New York, talking about health care ideas and about moving the foundation to Princeton. A few years later, we were all there together."

—ɯ— Beginnings

In December 1971, the Robert Wood Johnson Foundation officially opened its doors in a modest Victorian house in New Brunswick, New Jersey, with $1.2 billion in assets and the congressional requirement to spend $45 million in grants by the end of 1972. Gustav Lienhard, who had resigned as president of Johnson & Johnson on April 1, 1971, to become president and treasurer of the new foundation, was a crusty, no-nonsense businessman who announced his belief in "productive philanthropy."[3] David Rogers, formerly dean of the Johns Hopkins University School of Medicine, was named president as of January 1, 1972, while Lienhard became its full-time board chairman. Neither had ever worked for a foundation, much less one of the largest philanthropic institutions in the United States—second only to the Ford Foundation. Together, however, they assembled a remarkable team of health care experts that immediately forged new directions in the foundation world.

Keenan joined the Robert Wood Johnson Foundation as a senior executive associate in March 1972 (he was promoted to vice president later that year), based on the strong recommendation of Margaret Mahoney, who had been hired at the same time from the Carnegie Corporation to be a vice president at Robert Wood Johnson. ("As I remember it, Margaret said that she wouldn't come unless I went, and I wouldn't go unless she went," Keenan says. "So, happily, we went together.") Mahoney and Keenan were joined by Robert Blendon, who had worked with Rogers at Johns Hopkins and who is currently a professor of health policy at Harvard's School of Public Health, and Walsh McDermott, a physician and former chairman of the Department of Public Health at Cornell University Medical College. This quartet became Rogers's programmatic advisory group.

Because the staff was small at the beginning (twenty-one people are listed in the 1972 *Annual Report*), ideas were shared freely, and Rogers's style of leadership was casual. "We moved to the Forrestal campus at Princeton University soon after the Foundation was formed," recalls Ruby Hearn, who joined Robert Wood Johnson in 1976 as a program officer and retired in 2001 as senior vice president. "We were upstairs in the Forrestal Center, the same building as a linear accelerator. Almost every day, the entire staff, including Dr. Rogers, would have lunch around a common table. In that atmosphere, Terry Keenan was most effective because he could share his ideas quietly. Because of Terry's gentle manner, he was at risk of being underestimated in a larger forum. In that small group, we listened and learned. A lot of the ideas that became very important to the Foundation were originally suggested and nurtured by Terry. He was sort of the progenitor of many of the most significant programs we have ever done."[4]

Terry was deliberately unimposing. He used to dress almost every day in a white shirt, tie, slacks, and a wonderful tan windbreaker jacket that he would hang on a coat rack. He rarely wore a formal sport coat or a suit. He'd be at his desk, which was always piled high with papers, and start each day with a fresh yellow-lined pad and a half dozen freshly sharpened number-two pencils. He looked like how you might imagine one of the editors at the *New York Times*. He was a wordsmith and always found the right phrase, whether he was writing a presentation to the board or a memo to a colleague. Perhaps the most significant memory of Terry I have is that no matter how busy he was, he always made time to talk with a colleague.

—Alfred Sadler, former Robert Wood Johnson
Foundation assistant vice president

Although it would be unfair to attribute specific programs solely to any individual in a collective effort such as the Robert Wood Johnson Foundation in its early years, many of the fifty-seven grants listed in the 1972 *Annual Report* clearly reflect Keenan's career-long areas of passionate concern. For example, the largest grant authorization to a single institution in that first year, $5 million, went to Meharry Medical College in Nashville, Tennessee, to enlarge its primary care teaching facilities. At that time, Meharry graduated half of the nation's practicing African American physicians and 80 percent of those practicing in the thirteen Southern states. Margaret Mahoney's Clinical Scholars Program to train young physicians for leadership roles, which she had brought to Robert Wood Johnson from the Carnegie and Commonwealth foundations, received a $5.9 million grant. This is a program that Keenan had enthusiastically championed and worked on closely with Mahoney before they both joined the Robert Wood Johnson Foundation. A grant of $4 million for dental student aid again reflected Keenan's career emphasis on the need for greater access to dental health care.

Several smaller grants suggest programmatic areas that would later flourish under Keenan's care: a program at the University of California, Davis, to train rural nurse practitioners; a health care system study in Montgomery, Alabama; a network of rural health clinics near Provo, Utah; a summer study program in Newark, New Jersey, to prepare minority students to enter the health professions; and a grant to the Foundation Center for data collection and analysis of foundations. All were from Keenan's first Robert Wood Johnson portfolio.

Moving Ideas into the Mainstream

On the north bank of the Yukon River, about 470 miles northwest of Anchorage, Alaska, there is a remote fishing settlement, an enclave accessible only by dogsled and snowmobile in the winter, bush plane and small boats after the thaw.

At the hub of this village, just below the Arctic Circle, is a very modest health center. It is staffed by nine Yupik Inuits, who have been trained as community health aides. They speak halting English as a second language, but beam with pride as they describe the eighteen-week training program that transformed their lives and brought medical care to their frontier town.

Terry Keenan funded that training program in 1975. When I visited Mountain Village, Alaska, last week, I found that the model had been replicated among the frontier settlements that dot the Alaskan tundra. Moving an idea from the margins to the mainstream . . . that's Terry's forte. Terry also heralded nurse home visiting long before it was common. And there is no more genteel but dogged champion of nursing, midlevel professionals, training around domestic violence, services for the disabled, mobilizing volunteers for service, dental scholars, health care in public housing, minority student enrichment, early childhood literacy, parenting, and—of course—family centers.

—Judith Stavisky, Robert Wood Johnson
Foundation senior program officer

"Terry was originally brought into Robert Wood Johnson for internal management purposes rather than programmatic ideas," recalls former Foundation vice president Robert Blendon.

After all, he and Margaret Mahoney were the only ones with much real foundation experience. However, it very quickly became apparent that he had lots of valuable ideas about the role of foundations in general and about particular programs in health care. He held the strong view that a large foundation like ours could help to develop a network of small or medium-size foundations to share information; this eventually led to the formation of Grantmakers in Health. He also saw that funding at the community level was more effective when shared with other partners, which led to our Local Initiative Funding Partners Program. He perceived very early that many of the problems of health care had to do with shortages of nurses, the quality of nurse training, and the lack of leadership in the field. He made a very strong case for the value of faith-based health care programs, and argued that the Foundation should not be exclusively secular in its funding. He brought our attention to programs for dental health care, school-based adolescent health care, and other areas. But if I had to name Terry's greatest contribution to Robert Wood Johnson, it would be his relentless insistence that we never forget those vulnerable populations—elderly, disabled, children, minorities—who need health care in the inner cities and, most especially, all those small towns across America.

An examination of the astonishing 942 grants championed and supervised by Keenan supports Blendon's judgment. The grants in this portfolio have been made to numerous small community organizations all over the United States. A few are for millions of dollars and a few are for less than $10,000; most are for less than $100,000—modest by Robert Wood Johnson Foundation standards. Although Keenan's emphasis upon community initiatives, interfaith caregiving, school-based clinics, nursing, primary care for vulnerable populations, dental training, and services for disabled and elderly are well-represented, his commitments range across virtually every aspect of health and health care.

—〰— Local Initiative Funding Partners Program

From the beginning of Keenan's foundation career, he focused on community health care programs—particularly in small communities—and he quickly saw the need for a major reorganization of community funding practices. At the Ford Foundation and the Commonwealth Fund, he observed that local programs often disappeared after an initial three-year grant period. The grantees rarely made provisions for continued financial support. "The issue isn't what you can do about it, it's what you *have* to do about it," Keenan has observed. "You have to work on it and think about it and try to find ways to solve it. If you don't solve the problem, you can at least move the capacity to solve the problem more precisely and more vigorously ahead."[5]

Keenan set about finding a solution to the community health care problem through just the kind of inquiry he mentions. Rather than staying secure in the ivory tower of foundation offices, Keenan embarked on fact-finding missions in the field while simultaneously pursuing ways to partner with local philanthropic organizations. A trip to Texas in the late 1970s gave him a new insight into the problem. Journalist Irene Wielawski relates, "Keenan vividly remembers a trip to Texas, in which he called on foundations from one end of the state to the other trying to get them interested in financing a start-up health clinic in an abandoned church in San Antonio. . . . Keenan essentially acted as their ambassador."[6]

He failed in that effort. He was viewed as the voice of a big Yankee foundation that was not only meddling but also arrogant. Quite reasonably, local philanthropies wanted to know why, if the Robert Wood Johnson Foundation thought this health clinic was such a good idea, it didn't provide some funding. Chastened by his experience in Texas, Keenan realized that "it would be easier to get a favorable reception if I had some money to put on the table."

His earlier experimentation with funneling money into grassroots programs had resulted in the first community-based program of the Foundation, the Community Care Funding Partners Program, in the early 1980s. This program was characterized by its process: localized grant applications for school-based clinics and other primary care units had to satisfy a Foundation requirement for dollar-for-dollar matching funds from a local partnering funder. The idea was that the partnering institution would stay on and even help to gather additional funding after the Robert Wood Johnson Foundation's initial support ended. Frank Karel, former vice president of communications at the Foundation, called Keenan's idea "a stroke of genius," and noted, "No big foundation had ever done anything like this."

"I accompanied him on a site visit to Hazlehurst, Georgia, a small mill town in a rural community south of Macon," Peter Goodwin, the Foundation's vice president for national program affairs, recalls.

> I can't remember how long it took us to get there, but it seemed like forever. He had been there before, and they knew he was coming to discuss their plans for a community health center that he had funded through the Foundation. I thought we were meeting with two or three people. But when we rolled into town, you would have thought the president of the United States was arriving. I'd never in

my life seen such a spectacle. The whole town of about 350 people rolled out the red carpet for us. They literally closed down the town and took us to their country club, where the sheriff, who was attending, looked the other way about the local blue laws and joined in the toast to Terry Keenan. We were both embarrassed by this display of appreciation, but it was the most tangible evidence I've ever had that we are doing the right thing at the Foundation.

The full-scale Local Initiative Funding Partners program did not emerge until 1987, with a mandate to expand the scope of the Community Care Funding Partners program beyond funding for local clinics. The new entity gave considerable power to local philanthropies in selecting projects that they believed were deserving of support. Not surprisingly, many of the program's first grants dealt with such pressing but controversial social problems as child sex abuse, drug abuse, teen pregnancy, and HIV infection. At the center of the new program lay Keenan's sense of social responsibility. Musing on a foundation's *raison d'être,* he later remarked, "I think that foundations working with other entities at the local, state, but also the national level can use their funds not only for convening but for looking at issues and understanding problems. If you go back to what foundation philanthropy represents in our society, it really is the principal source of private development capital investing in social purposes."[7]

Despite giving local voices a hearing, however, there were internal problems with the plan at the Foundation. According to Irene Wielawski, "It stood out as a radical departure from the status quo, and discomfort within the staff was palpable."[8] In response to internal pressures as well as a curtailment of grantmaking in general, the program was shut down in 1989, at the end of its second round of funding.

But Keenan did not give up; he adopted a ruminative position instead. Pauline Seitz, current director of the Local Initiative Funding Partners program, recalls, "Terry never hesitated to just roll over, pretending he was dead. . . . It was sort of a turtle technique that Terry had. He would just get bombarded and critiqued from all sides, and he'd sort of go into his shell . . . and when nobody was looking he'd just crawl out very slowly and proceed back on course, and he'd inevitably get across the finish line."

I had just concluded a wonderful job interview with Terry for a job as program officer for Local Initiative Funding Partners program in August of 1987 and we were waiting for my next interviewer to be available. He looked out of his office, across the atrium to the other offices in the building and seemed to be lost in thought for a moment. He turned to me and said, "You know, working here isn't for everybody. The Foundation is sort of like the Wizard of Oz, and you have to stay behind the curtain. You have to understand that the most significant work of the organization is done by the grantees. We are simply the agents of their success, and they deserve the credit. If you have a need for direct recognition, it can be a very frustrating environment, because everything that happens here takes place behind the mask of that Wizard called the Robert Wood Johnson Foundation."

—Pauline Seitz, director of the Local Initiative
Funding Partners program

Steven Schroeder recalls that when he became president of the Robert Wood Johnson Foundation, in 1990, he felt an almost immediate kinship with Keenan. "One of the first things I did when I moved into the Foundation offices was to place on my desk a quotation sent to me by my friend, John Kenneth Galbraith," Schroeder says. "It reads, 'Nothing so gives the illusion of intelligence as a personal association with large sums of money.' Terry liked that quote, and he helped me to guard against Foundation arrogance by his example and by the occasional quiet comment."

Before his appointment, Schroeder candidly informed the board of the Robert Wood Johnson Foundation that he intended to lead the Foundation in a more active role to combat the social roots of health care problems in America. One of his first acts was to reinstate the Local Initiative Funding Partners program. "Terry's program was central to how I thought the Foundation should operate," Schroeder recalls. "It permitted us to have an ear to the ground all throughout the country; to work through others; to honor those others; to be a senior but equal partner; and to respect people. It is a great grassroots program." As Schroeder recalls, there was still internal resistance when he revived the program, and Keenan was "not a glamorous salesman, but he was a tenacious salesman. Ultimately, I think all of our staff became very proud of that program."[9]

In a memorandum of October 24, 1990, to Schroeder, Keenan suggested some new rules to address a problem that faced the Local Initiative program. The Foundation had been requiring its local foundation partners to guarantee that matching funds would be made available, even before the Foundation had itself agreed to fund a project. This created resentments since, as Irene Wielawski has written, "Qualifying for the Foundation match translated into months of effort, including personal and public advocacy. . . . The design flaw was potentially fatal to the Foundation's goal of genuine partnership with communities."[10] Keenan recommended that the Foundation drop the controversial requirement that partner-funders guarantee matching funds *before* the Robert Wood Johnson Foundation made a commitment—a recommendation that was accepted. Today, local funders are simply asked for a statement of intention instead of a guarantee of matching funds.

"The Local Initiative Funding Partners Program was an outstanding contribution," Schroeder points out. "Terry nurtured it at a time when it wasn't that popular. Now it is part of the Foundation's DNA."

—〰— Interfaith Caregiving

Perhaps no other program exemplifies Terry Keenan's strong sense of coalition building better than the Foundation's interfaith partnership efforts. Keenan is a man of strong spiritual beliefs, and he keeps them private. From his earliest days at the Foundation, Keenan saw the value of partnering with hospitals, community medical centers, and local organizations that were faith-based. Understandably, there was considerable opposition within the Foundation to the appearance of financing religious institutions. After a decade of making small grants, the Foundation committed to a major initiative in 1983 with a $2.3 million grant to the fledgling Interfaith Volunteer Caregivers Program. The funding would provide three-year grants of $50,000 a year to fifteen churches, synagogues, and other houses of worship in fifteen communities around the country to set up coalitions where members of their different faith communities would provide care—such as transportation to doctors' offices, shopping, and companionship—to chronically ill people.

The Interfaith Caregivers Program was clearly a test of Keenan's conviction that a health services foundation should help tackle day-to-day issues of chronic care along with more traditional health services—and could do so by fostering partnerships of religious organizations. He recognized that "It should be possible to foster common purpose among institutions with similar missions—service to youth, for example—without loss of individual identity."[11] He identified this sense of common purpose in the general call to service that is part of the religious doctrine of many faiths. But he realized that within the well-intentioned efforts of most churches or synagogues lay the possibility of redundancy of effort. If the Foundation could foster interfaith programs sharing resources and person power, the crying need for volunteer caregiving could be harnessed and focused.

The initial announcement of the program was met by more than a thousand letters of intent from organizations all over the country. In response, the Foundation increased the number of sites from ten to twenty-five. Under the aegis of Kenneth Johnson, an internist at Kingston Hospital in Kingston, New York, and director of its health services research center, a demonstration program was launched with twenty-five interfaith coalitions. Johnson had worked closely with several previous Foundation programs. The money supported a paid director to coordinate and direct the volunteer efforts of these religious organizations. The rationale for paid directors stemmed from the idea that a paid staff person could better structure the enterprise, organize volunteers, and continually revise and adapt the plan for caregiving than a council of representatives, who might meet only sporadically. Many of the locations and other auxiliary supplies were provided by member denominations. Johnson observed, "Interfaith volunteer caregiver programs fill gaps in the long-term care system."[12]

The fact that ten years later, twenty of the initial twenty-five interfaith groups were still in existence testified not only to the need but also to the viability of these groups working together. Such was the positive response that in 1993 the Foundation invited interfaith caregiving organizations to submit applications for a new program, called Faith in Action, that replicated and expanded the concept. The program's supporters envisioned making enough grants so that eventually an interfaith coalition could exist in almost every corner of the United States.[13]

Each location needed to exhibit certain features, including:

- An authentic interfaith or ecumenical governance, involving a broad spectrum of faiths and denominations working together
- An average number of fifty volunteers serving fifty persons during the first twelve months of the program
- Volunteer caregiving that was direct, person-to-person, and hands-on, and that provided multiple kinds of assistance rather than a single service

Technical assistance was provided by twelve federation-sponsored regional facilitators, who were to help the coalitions make applications, build the coalitions, and secure matching funds and other administrative services.

Under the second round of funding for Faith in Action, 1,091 interfaith coalitions received Foundation support. In July 1998, when the last of the second-round grants had been awarded, nearly 60,000 people were volunteering their services under Faith in Action, or an average of fifty-seven volunteers per site.

In September 1999, the Foundation approved a third generation of the Faith in Action program. The retooled program, which sought to distribute $100 million to two thousand new faith-based coalitions over a seven-year period, was intended to expand its reach by coordinating with heretofore untraditional organizations such as the National Council of La Raza and the Islamic Society of North America. Features included grants of $35,000 per site, more technical support, and a new computer network that links coalitions and pools a variety of online resources.

In 2004, the Foundation decided to make final funding authorization to the program and to concentrate its resources on other initiatives.

Nonetheless, Faith in Action is considered by many as a signature program of the Foundation. The credit, former Foundation vice president Paul Jellinek says, goes to Terry Keenan: "He was at the forefront of the interfaith caregiving movement, which started with a small demonstration program that Terry pushed through the Foundation back in 1983. The Robert Wood Johnson Foundation has now supported 1,100 of these coalitions around the country. It all goes back to Terry and his feelings about impact and scale."

—⬩— Nurses' Training; Physician's Assistants; Emergency Medical Services

"Nurturing, caring, healing—that's what drives nursing, that caring sense," Keenan says. "It is really the ethos of the profession. I am very proud that the Foundation has taken a leadership role in the development of nursing, expanding the content of nursing, building up the education of nurses, and supporting the concept of the nurse practitioner. One of my first projects at the Foundation was to support nursing schools, particularly at the graduate level. To my amazement, a lot of people—including some of the deans of these schools—disagreed with that idea [graduate-level nurse practitioners]."

"It is strange to recall how controversial all the issues around nurses and nurse practitioners were at the beginning," says Ruby Hearn, former Robert Wood Johnson Foundation senior vice president. "Doctors were upset about the financial aspects of their roles and what medical functions nurses might be authorized to perform. Terry was particularly supportive of clinics run by free-standing nurse practitioners, and that was extremely controversial. Of course, today, the expanded role of nurses and nurse practitioners is considered an absolutely necessary part of the medical establishment."

As with so many of Keenan's ideas, his concepts about nursing—including an expanded role for nurses, specialized medical training for nurses and physician's assistants, restructuring of hospital nursing care, use of emergency registered nurses in remote rural areas, and clinics headed by nurse practitioners—were considered revolutionary in the 1970s.[14]

"My brother Blair and I first met Terry Keenan in the summer of 1970 at the Commonwealth Fund, in that beautiful old building of theirs on the corner of 75th Street and Central Park," recalls Alfred Sadler, a former Robert Wood Johnson Foundation assistant vice president. "The Fund had just granted $2 million for a very imaginative program in emergency medicine and trauma management under the direction of Jack Cole, who was chairman of surgery at the Yale School of Medicine."[15] Blair and Alfred Sadler, identical twins, were hired to run this program, and they quickly convinced Cole that Yale should sponsor a program for physician's assistants in emergency care that was similar to the pioneering Duke University Physician Assistant program in general medicine under Eugene Stead.

"During our three years at Yale, Fred and I stayed in close communication with Terry at Commonwealth and Maggie Mahoney at Carnegie," says Blair Sadler, who is also a former Robert Wood Johnson Foundation assistant vice president. "In fact, they supported us and encouraged us to write *The Physician's Assistant—Today and Tomorrow* (Yale University Press, 1972) with a colleague at Yale, Ann Bliss. This was a summary of the work we had done and of the developments in the field at that point. To give you an illustration of how closely we worked together, that book is dedicated to Terry and Maggie."

In 1973, David Rogers, then the president of the Robert Wood Johnson Foundation, came to Yale to give a speech and met the Sadlers. After that meeting and some discussions with Keenan and Mahoney, who were already at the Robert Wood Johnson Foundation, Rogers invited the Sadlers to join the Foundation and to take their successful Yale Emergency Medical Services program nationwide. "We couldn't believe the collegial atmosphere at the Foundation headquarters in Princeton," Blair Sadler recalls. "The entire staff would sit around a lunch table and dream about how to solve the health care problems of the United States. Terry never dominated these casual meetings, but when he spoke everyone listened carefully, because he always had insights and ideas that were based on his experiences in the field. He was passionate about the need for training and utilizing physician assistants and nurse practitioners."

"From those early days to the present, Terry Keenan's achievements have been remarkable," Alfred Sadler says. "But more than that, his influence, his personality, and his thinking about grantmaking have been hugely influential in the whole world of philanthropy, especially in medical and health care foundations. His humanistic approach, his willingness to take risks, or even fail, and his concern that foundations have to look to the future—Terry has changed foundation culture for the better by his example."

Although Keenan has always credited many Robert Wood Johnson Foundation colleagues for their important contributions—including Margaret Mahoney, the Sadlers, Linda Aiken, Ruby Hearn, and Nancy Kaufman—there is no doubt that he took the initiative in advancing multiple changes in the world of nursing. "Terry was very committed to school-based clinics when I arrived at the Foundation in 1972," recalls Edward Robbins, former director of the office of proposal management at the Foundation. "The area was controversial for many reasons. First, it was a new area for the Foundation, which had been accustomed to working with hospitals and universities. Second, religious and political organizations objected to nurses providing birth control information to adolescents. And, third, doctors were uncomfortable with the expanded diagnostic role nurses were playing in these schools. Quite frankly, in many cases, the nurses were taking more initiative about the children's health care than the parents were."

Some of the grants in Keenan's 1972 portfolio included funding for a nurse practitioner program for rural areas that was supervised by the new Department of Family Practice at the University of California, Davis, and training for nurse practitioners at the Utah Valley Hospital in Provo. Keenan championed grants to the Tuskegee Institute in Alabama in 1973 and 1974 to utilize teams of nurse practitioners working from a mobile van to make an initial assessment of the health needs of families in a three-county area of Alabama; in 1974, he convinced the Foundation to provide funding for Kentucky's Frontier Nursing Service to develop a curriculum for training of family nurse practitioners; and in that same year he recommended a grant to Adelphi University in Garden City, New York, to study the role of nurses in primary care. By 1978, the Foundation, based on Keenan's recommendations, had funded more than a dozen nurse and physician's assistant training programs around the country. These included the Program to Equip Emergency Nurses with Primary Care Skills to train emergency room nurses from small regional hospitals in six university-affiliated hospitals, and the School Health Services Program, which brought nurse practitioners to 150,000 children of low-income parents in thirty-six urban elementary schools, and which was the first of a number of Foundation-funded school-based health programs.

A lot of people at foundations are basically academics. They don't like to get their hands dirty or to come out of the ivory tower. Well, Terry was just the opposite. For example, in 1988, he heard about a program for poor children in Chicago called Project Beethoven. As always, he didn't just pick up the telephone. He got on the plane to Chicago. So here is Terry, by this time in his career an older gentleman and a little frail from just having had cardiac bypass surgery, going into the worst neighborhood in the South Side of Chicago. It was extremely rough at the time. Mothers were afraid to allow their children to play on the playgrounds. There was crack cocaine addiction and people shooting at each other every day. You could get killed just getting out of a taxicab in this neighborhood. Here comes gray-haired Terry, all by himself, walking down the block, trying to find the right address. People from the project looked out of a second-story window and saw him picking his way over piles of trash. They ran down the stairs to get him.

His hosts told me that they were horrified when he arrived alone. But he put them at ease. He sat down with them and listened to their problems. He went into the classrooms and met the children. Then he came back to the Foundation and wrote a million-dollar grant to build a health clinic and to develop a coordinated plan to link the public health nursing, social services, and educational services for the children. From there, Terry went on to create a whole child development initiative for the country. He brought in other foundations and showed them how to replicate this model of providing sanctuaries for children within very bad neighborhoods. He basically revolutionized the field, and today there are hundreds of child development centers all over the country based on the ideas he initiated at Beethoven.

—Nancy Kaufman, former vice president at the Robert Wood Johnson Foundation

The Foundation has continued to support the field of nursing, including the $7 million Teaching Nursing Home Program, the $11 million Clinical Nurse Scholars Program, the $17 million program for Strengthening Hospital Nursing, the $29.7 million Executive Nurse Fellows Program, and the $1.8 million Transforming Care at the Bedside Program. Nurse practitioners and physician assistants have become a recognized part of America's health care system. The Foundation has given more than $140 million to nursing programs, and continues its strong commitment to the field.[16]

—w— Grantmakers in Health

Almost from the moment Terry Keenan arrived at the Foundation, he began networking with other foundations. He shared information about the activities of the Robert Wood Johnson Foundation and, in many cases, attempted to coordinate funding of programs. There were a limited number of philanthropies in the United States that were working on health issues, and Keenan was aware that they never sat down at a table together to discuss common problems or to learn from one another. For more than a decade, he acted as a one-man communications center among the health care foundations, until he was able to create a national organization called Grantmakers in Health in 1982.

Grantmakers in Health now brings together some 330 foundations and corporate grantmaking organizations in a regular series of meetings, workshops, issue-focused forums, and publications about health and health care issues. Since 1998, it also has operated the Resource Center on Health Philanthropy, which collects data from health philanthropies and identifies trends in the field. As a tribute to his importance in the field, the Terrance Keenan Leadership Award in Health Philanthropy is presented by Grantmakers in Health every year to an outstanding individual in the field. "We feel that this award recognizes Mr. Keenan's importance in health philanthropy, and regularly reminds us of his values and spirit," says Lauren LeRoy, president and chief executive officer of Grantmakers in Health.

—w— An Appreciation

"Terry's heartfelt compassion for the most vulnerable in our society came across in the way he approached philanthropy," Risa Lavizzo-Mourey, president and CEO of the Foundation, said in a speech honoring Keenan last year. "When Terry joined the Robert Wood Johnson Foundation, foundations in general were not terribly active; they did not have a mission and a program for change. In fact, philanthropy was considered suspect by many people who believed wealthy individuals were establishing foundations to use as tax write-offs. Terry helped change both the reality and the perception of foundations." In that same speech, she said, "Describing someone as a 'legend' may seem excessive. But in the case of Terrance Keenan, the term is entirely appropriate."

Notes

1. Keenan, T. *The Promise at Hand.* Princeton, N.J.: Robert Wood Johnson Foundation Publications, 1992. Unpublished revised manuscript, 2003.
2. Jellinek, P. Speech at Grantmakers in Health, Terrance Keenan Award luncheon, March 2, 2000, Miami, Fla.
3. Pace University Web site. Gustav O. Lienhard biography. (http://webpage.pace.edu/mweigold/lienhardbio.html).
4. Interview with Ruby Hearn, November 20, 2004.
5. Keenan, T. Speech at Grantmakers in Health Awards ceremonies, March 2, 2000, Miami, Fla.
6. Wielawski, I. M. "The Local Initiative Funding Partners Program." *To Improve Health and Health Care, 2000: The Robert Wood Johnson Foundation Anthology.* San Francisco: Jossey-Bass, 1999.
7. Keenan, T. Grantmakers in Health Awards ceremonies, 2000.
8. Wielawski, p. 162.
9. Ibid.
10. Ibid.
11. Keenan, T. Preface. *Reflections on Grantmaking.* (http://www.rwjf.org/library/reflect7.htm.)
12. Faith in Action National Program Report, updated April 2004. (http://www.rwjf.org/reports/nreports/faithinaction.htm).
13. Jellinek, P., Gibbs Appel, T., Keenan, T. "Faith in Action." *To Improve Health and Health Care 1998–1999: The Robert Wood Johnson Foundation Anthology.* San Francisco: Jossey-Bass, 1998.
14. Keenan, T. "Support of Nurse Practitioners and Physician Assistants." *To Improve Health and Health Care 1998–1999: The Robert Wood Johnson Foundation Anthology.* San Francisco: Jossey-Bass, 1998.
15. Diehl, D. "The Emergency Medical Services Program." *To Improve Health and Health Care 1998–1999: The Robert Wood Johnson Foundation Anthology.* San Francisco: Jossey-Bass, 1998.
16. Newbergh, C. "The Robert Wood Johnson Foundation's Commitment to Nursing." *To Improve Health and Health Care, Vol. VIII: The Robert Wood Johnson Foundation Anthology.* San Francisco: Jossey-Bass, 2005.

Issues in Philanthropy

Public Scrutiny of Foundations and Charities

The Robert Wood Johnson Foundation Response

Susan Krutt and David Morse[1]

Editors' Introduction

American foundations are a unique national resource, serving as stewards of private resources used in the public interest. Responsible primarily to their own boards of directors—as contrasted with, say, the electorate or shareholders—foundations are, in the words of Alan Pifer, former president of the Carnegie Corporation of New York, "the least constrained of all institutions in our society."[2] Unlike most other institutions, foundations have a dual public and private nature. They are private corporations whose endowments come from wealthy individuals and corporations. Under the Internal Revenue Code, the income on foundations' investments is largely tax-exempt.

Given foundations' lack of public accountability and the importance of the tax exemption to their very existence—not to mention their reputation for being secretive—it is not surprising that the federal government scrutinizes foundations to make sure that they use their resources legally and, at least arguably, for purposes that benefit the public. Nor is it surprising—in light of the recent highly publicized corporate and nonprofit organization scandals—that Congress would single out foundations for special attention at this time.

In this chapter, Susan Krutt, a communications associate at the Robert Wood Johnson Foundation, and David Morse, the Foundation's vice president for communications, provide an overview of congressional scrutiny of foundations and charitable organizations and the sector's response. They place the recent Senate hearings in the context of past congressional examinations of foundations, analyze the underlying issues, and explain how philanthropy is trying to address concerns about its lack of accountability. The authors conclude by discussing the approaches adopted by the Robert Wood Johnson Foundation to make its own work more transparent, especially through its evaluation and communications strategies.

---

1. The authors express their appreciation to Katherine Hatton, Carol Kroch, and James Ingram for their insightful review of this chapter.
2. Pifer, A. *Speaking Out: Reflections on 30 Years of Foundation Work.* Washington, D.C.: Council on Foundations, 2001.

Ouch! For charities that see themselves as beneficent social problem solvers and integral to a national spirit of generosity, the spate of headlines in some of America's leading newspapers hurt, and hurt badly: "CEO's Rewards at Nonprofit," "Costly Furnishings Come at Charities' Expense," "Philanthropist's Millions Enrich Family Retainers," "Wealthiest Nonprofits Favored by Foundations," "Nonprofit on Trial for Its Excess," "IRS Chief Says Nonprofits Are Vulnerable to Abuses." Beginning with a series of stories in the *San Jose Mercury News* in the spring of 2003, America's philanthropies, unaccustomed to and uncomfortable being in the public spotlight except to be appreciated for their benevolence, have increasingly found their *bona fides* questioned, both individually and collectively as a sector, with an intensity not felt for more than thirty years. The stories were more reminiscent of investigations uncovering recent scandals and abuses in large for-profit corporations like Enron, Tyco, and WorldCom than of the typical reporting of "good works" performed by America's nonprofit sector.

The headlines captured the attention of policymakers, most notably state attorneys general across the country as well as members of Congress with oversight of the federal tax laws that regulate charitable activities. Congress's focus was less on foundations *per se* than on apparent abuses and complex tax scams festering throughout the larger charitable sector, including gross overvaluations of gifts of property, such as conservation easements and cars, to sometimes complacent and complicit charities.

For example, during a break in a standing-room-only hearing room in June 2004, Senate Finance Committee members and hearing attendees watched as an opaque screen was pulled out onto the floor in preparation for testimony from two anonymous witnesses. Known only as "Mr. Car" and "Mr. House," they proceeded to speak from behind the screen, through a voice-modifying device, blowing the whistle on complex schemes led by organizations that were stealing millions of dollars from Americans who thought they had made legitimate charitable gifts.

As the mechanized voices echoed through the room, members of the audience raised eyebrows and exchanged whispers. This, after all, was high drama for a hearing on the nation's charities—the sector that has been considered, since the days of De Tocqueville, the cornerstone of America's altruistic and voluntary spirit.

Indeed, Mr. Car and Mr. House got their names because they blew the whistle on nonprofit organizations that used the guise of charity to rip people off. Mr. Car had witnessed the brokering of donated cars to charitable groups, and Mr. House's testimony exposed an organization that helped low-income Americans afford down payments on home purchases. According to Mr. Car, donors assumed they were contributing the full value of their vehicles but ultimately the charities received less than 10 percent of that amount. The executives Mr. House described issued contracts to related groups that lined their own pockets with the proceeds.

Mr. Car and Mr. House disclosed two, but by no means the only two, cases of charitable malfeasance, and members of the Finance Committee seemed prepared to recommend a sweeping set of legislative reforms to increase and enforce compliance with regulations, restore public trust and accountability, and instill strong governance measures across America's charitable sector.

By the end of the summer of 2004, charities wondered whether they were about to be taken to the woodshed simply because a few bad actors had tarnished their otherwise virtuous sector, or whether the entire charitable enterprise had gone seriously astray. There was genuine cause for concern; although there have always been exceptions, foundations and other charities have generally served the public good and stayed well within the boundaries of legal, ethical, and accountable practice. In the past decade, however, there has been a notable upswing in public attention to, and regulatory scrutiny of, mismanagement and malfeasance among America's nonprofit organizations. The upshot? An erosion of the public trust that is vested in charities and that is the rationale for their tax exemption and the corollary tax deduction for charitable donations.

Senate Finance Committee Chairman Chuck Grassley opened the June 2004 hearing by describing that trust relationship: "Today the Finance Committee considers a very serious matter: ensuring that charities keep their trust with the American people. We will hear testimony today that is troubling, very troubling, suggesting that far too many charities have broken the understood covenant between the taxpayer and the non-profits. That covenant is that charities are to benefit the public good, not fill the pockets of private individuals."[1]

Foundations—a relatively small but influential segment of the non-profit world—were not exempt from the critique or the purported cure. Finance Committee members questioned foundations' grantmaking and accounting practices, executive compensation levels, and trustee governance practices, and called for foundation-specific reforms at the hearing. On the heels of the Senate hearing, the Internal Revenue Service announced that it would investigate executive compensation packages at nearly two thousand charities and audit about four hundred foundations as part of a sweeping effort to heighten accountability and weed out bad practices.[2]

Other proposed oversight measures also would shake up philanthropies. The Senate Finance Committee considered a proposal to have the IRS review organizations' tax-exempt status every five years and have groups with $250,000 or more in gross receipts submit independent audits of financial statements, and held a second hearing, in April 2005, to reassess the need for legislative and regulatory action to promote integrity among nonprofits. Some state regulators reached even further. On January 1, 2005, California's Nonprofit Integrity Act went into effect requiring all charities to have their boards review and approve "just and reasonable" executive compensation, groups with gross revenues over $2 million to have independent audits, and commercial fundraisers to register new solicitation campaigns with the attorney general.[3] And in Minnesota, legislators introduced a bill in February 2005 requiring any nonprofit receiving state funds and paying employees salaries that exceed the governor's compensation ($120,303) to supply the attorney general with a list of salaries for its three highest-paid staff members. A related measure would make charities in this category list compensation totals for their three highest-paid directors, officers, or employees on all fundraising materials.[4]

These days, regulators are tracking foundation practices more vigorously as well, and they are quick to punish abusive or unethical practices. In 2004, in a suit brought by the Texas attorney general, a jury ordered three leaders of the Carl B. and Florence E. King Foundation to repay, in total, more than $20 million to the foundation that they received in salaries, benefit packages, and other perks.[5] In California, the president of the James Irvine Foundation and his wife repaid the foundation more than $30,000 for a parting gift that was found to be illegal and to rectify a self-dealing charge stemming from the wife's occasional use of Irvine's facilities to operate her consulting firm.[6]

The Nonprofit Sector

The organizations discussed in this chapter are all part of the "third" or "independent" nonprofit sector of the economy—that is, the sector that is neither government nor business. Discussion of the nonprofit sector can be confusing, in part because of the bewildering complexity of the nonprofit sector itself and in part because of the tendency of commentators to conflate the terms *nonprofit* and *tax exempt* with *charity*. While all charities are nonprofits, not all nonprofits are charities. In fact, the Internal Revenue Code lists twenty-eight categories of nonprofit organizations that are exempt from federal income taxes, including social welfare organizations, trade associations, fraternal organizations, social clubs, and veterans' organizations, among others. However, only one category of nonprofit organization—those organized exclusively for religious, charitable (including health), scientific, literary, or educational purposes—are *charities* entitled to receive tax deductible contributions. (Charities are sometimes referred to as 501(c)(3)'s after the section of the Internal Revenue Code that defines them.) This chapter is concerned with charities and to a lesser extent social welfare organizations, but not the rest of the nonprofit sector.

Most charities solicit funds from and/or provide charitable or educational services to the general public. This group includes churches, hospitals, colleges and universities, museums, and publicly supported voluntary organizations, such as the United Way, Red Cross, American Heart Association, and American Cancer Society. These organizations are widely known and for the most part admired in their communities.

There is a smaller, less visible class of charitable organizations known generally as *foundations,* which generally do not provide services directly to the public, but instead carry out their charitable missions primarily by making grants to other charities. Foundations, as the term is used here, include private foundations and community foundations. Private foundations can be funded by a small group of individuals or can be corporate foundations that are funded by and carry out the charitable activities of a particular company. On the other hand, community foundations manage multiple funds contributed by multiple donors. Both private and community foundations solicit funds and make grants, and most are classified as public charities by the IRS.

Because private foundations operate largely outside the public eye, they are less known to the general public than are other charities. A 2003 survey of the public and policymakers conducted by Wirthlin Worldwide found that when asked to name a foundation, more than half of survey respondents did not know of any or did not respond, and 12 percent named a publicly supported charity like the United Way or the Red Cross.[7] However, because foundation grants are an important source of funds to other charities, foundations are widely known within the nonprofit sector. This chapter focuses to a significant extent on the particular role and concerns of grantmaking foundations and their relationship to government, to the public, and to those charities that are the recipients of grants and provide charitable services to the public.

For definitions of the technical or legal terms used in this chapter, see the glossary at the end of the chapter.

—〰— Regulatory Action and Philanthropic Reaction

These are but recent episodes in a drama that has been playing out, with occasional intermissions, for nearly a century. At the 1916 Walsh Commission hearings, which investigated whether foundations held too much influence over the nation's economic, educational, and social spheres, some critics berated the philanthropic pioneers Andrew Carnegie and John D. Rockefeller for designating what the appropriate "objects of philanthropy" should be. Liberal populists, labor leaders, and others believed this was something the American people, through public institutions, should decide for themselves.[8]

Over the last forty to fifty years—while the foundation world as we know it has taken shape—several periods of legislative inquiry have shaken the stability of the nonprofit sector. Across most all of these inquiries, certain themes recur: distrust of foundations as private, influential, but unaccountable pools of wealth; tension over the allocation of funds directly supporting charitable works versus internal administrative costs; and the appropriate role of foundations and their philanthropic benefactors in public policymaking. Indeed, the pattern of legislative and regulatory review has been cyclical, driven by familiar critiques of charitable organizations' behavior. Two widely held premises have driven the debates over the role of philanthropy in general and foundations in particular: the expectation that philanthropists should marshal private wealth to benefit the public good, and the tax exemptions and deductions that derive from that expectation.

The 1960s and the Tax Reform Act of 1969

The social upheaval of the 1960s presented the backdrop for several grantmakers to participate in political and civil rights debates. Some foundations—most notably the Ford Foundation, the nation's largest at that time—were deeply engaged in fostering social movements, tackling root causes as well as symptoms of urban poverty and racial inequality. When Ford gave Cleveland's Congress on Racial Equality and the Southern Regional Council grant funds to stage voter registration drives, several political leaders cried foul, charging that a tax-exempt foundation should not be allowed to use private funds to sway elections. In addition to the activism of some foundations, the 1960s saw an increase in the sheer number of foundations. New philanthropies were registered at the rate of 1,200 a year; some disregarded their core public benefit obligation by serving as little more than tax shelters for the affluent. Representative Wright Patman, a populist Democrat from Texas, viewed these as untaxed silos of private wealth, often established in perpetuity. In 1961, Patman opened an eight-year probe of foundations. Although the Treasury Department's 1965 *Report on Private Foundations* concluded that most foundations served a beneficial social purpose and did not abuse the tax system, it also reinforced several of Patman's concerns: some foundations were used for improper private gain, had inappropriate business holdings, or stockpiled money rather than granting it to charitable recipients.

Foundations were on the defensive, and it was unclear how hard Congress would crack down on the field. New regulation could have been stifling: Senator Albert Gore Sr., concerned about perpetuity, wanted to forbid any foundation to operate for more than twenty-five years. Although Patman's legacy, the Tax Reform Act of 1969, stripped away some of the more drastic proposals such as Gore's, it included landmark provisions regulating private foundation practices. It created a legal distinction between public charities—often educational institutions, churches, hospitals, and United Way–type organizations so classified because of their activities or because they receive a substantial amount of support from the general public and government—and private foundations, which do not meet the activity or public support test. Most foundations are classified as private foundations under the Act, although some, such as community foundations, have sufficient public support to be considered public charities.

The Tax Reform Act imposed a series of regulatory restrictions on private foundations that do not apply to public charities. Among them were

- Setting a minimum payout level that required a private foundation to spend a minimum of 6 percent of its assets or all net investment income each year, whichever was greater. In 1981, Congress reduced this level to 5 percent and eliminated the alternate calculation.

- Levying a 4 percent net excise tax—later dropped to 2 percent—on net investment income, including capital gains. The tax falls to 1 percent if certain requirements are met.

- Prohibiting lobbying, except for "self-defense" lobbying on legislative matters that affect the foundation's legal or tax status. Lobbying also does not include broad discussion of social issues and nonpartisan analysis, study, and research—work that permits foundations to support or do significant public policy work.

- Placing strict conditions on voter registration grants, supplementing the existing prohibitions on all charities against intervention in political campaigns.

- Barring foundations from holding more than 20 percent of a business enterprise, including stock in a corporation or interest in a partnership.

- Instituting a ban on self-dealing, generally defined as direct or indirect financial transactions between a foundation and its trustees, officers, donors, and their family members. An exception permits a foundation to pay "reasonable compensation" for personal services provided to it.

- Prohibiting excessively risky investments.

- Expanding the tax return that foundations must make available for public inspection.

- Enforcing all of these prohibitions through a series of excise taxes, so that revocation of the foundation's tax-exempt status is no longer the only penalty available to regulators.[9]

The 1969 Tax Reform Act remains the most sweeping act of legislation to affect the nonprofit and philanthropic sectors. Its effects continue to guide foundations' behavior in powerful ways to the present day.

The 1970s

With the Tax Reform Act in place, private foundations entered the 1970s knowing that they could no longer fly unseen under the radar of government regulators. A new commission established in 1970 and chaired by John Gardner, former president of the Carnegie Corporation of New York, explored how grantmakers could rebuild public trust in their work and prevent future punitive regulation. The Commission on Private Philanthropy and Public Needs, more commonly called the Filer Commission after its chairman, John H. Filer, the chief executive officer of Aetna, followed soon thereafter. Beginning in 1973, it undertook the task of analyzing both the role of philanthropy in America and the universe of charitable, or "voluntary," organizations that receive foundation funds. Two years later, Commission members outlined their vision for how charities and "the practice of private giving" could be improved.

Although it did not lead to new legislation, the Filer Commission spurred several critical developments within philanthropy. For the first time, grantors and grantees came to think of themselves as part of the same overarching, independent sector. Philanthropists and grantees acknowledged their shared strengths, together with their governance and accountability hurdles. A subgroup of grantees involved in the commission went on to form the National Committee for Responsive Philanthropy, or NCRP, the first watchdog group to monitor the policies and principles of grantmaking foundations.

Within five years, the legacy of the Filer Commission produced Independent Sector, a central membership and advocacy group for America's voluntary sector. Independent Sector joined NCRP, the Council on Foundations (philanthropy's national trade association), the Foundation Center (the leading data repository on foundations), other national organizations in a broader effort to define and promote the value of foundations and other charities in society, and, if necessary, to be the advocates for the sector's interests and its tax exemption.

Philanthropies and other charities in the independent sector were beginning to build an infrastructure to promote stronger understanding among policymakers and the public of their distinct role and impact. While those who had gone through the battles of the 1960s hoped that such efforts would prevent further regulatory upheaval, sector leaders had learned that they had better be prepared for future inquiries into their operations.

The 1980s and 1990s

Regulatory attention to private foundations decreased somewhat in the 1980s and 1990s. In the early eighties, the IRS completed an "examination study" of private foundations and cited high overall compliance with federal requirements, prompting fewer audits of funders. Testifying before the Senate Finance Committee in 2004, IRS Commissioner Mark Everson pointed to this long-standing compliance as a chief reason that regulatory audits of tax-exempt groups had been relatively infrequent.[10] During the 1990s, grantmakers primarily rallied around preserving and defending the advocacy responsibilities and rights of their nonprofit grantees, which came under assault by some in Congress. In 1995, Oklahoma Republican Representative Ernest Istook and two other congressmen introduced an amendment that would have limited the ability of nonprofits that received federal grants or contracts to use privately raised funds to educate Congress, influence policy, or otherwise speak out on legislation.

Istook amendment supporters framed the issue as one of federally supported nonprofits misusing tax-exempt public dollars—an injustice to taxpayers that had to be stopped. A diverse set of funders and charities rallied around the proposition that advocacy is fundamental to nonprofits' role in American democracy, and that the use of private funds for advocacy should be safeguarded, not chilled. The Istook amendment failed, but it served up a strong reminder to nonprofit leaders who may have forgotten the precariousness of their regulatory standing.

—w— An Accountability Crisis? Is Transparency the Solution?

Since 2001, policymakers have been consumed with governance and accountability scandals that cut a wide swath across major American institutions: corporations, government, even the church. The most notorious offenders are corporate giants whose leaders placed their own interests ahead of shareholders, employees, and customers. This has shaken public trust in institutions throughout society; by extension, it is not surprising to see private foundations and public charities—those organizations charged with fostering public good with private means—called to account as well. Paul Light, a professor of public service at New York University and nonresident senior fellow at the Brookings Institution, verifies this trend. His research indicates that confidence in America's charities nosedived after September 11th, when many Americans disapproved of the way charitable organizations such as the Red Cross managed the allocation of donations raised in response to the terrorist attacks. Confidence levels still stand 10 to 15 percent lower than they did in the summer of 2001.[11] And, speaking in April 2005 to the Council on Foundations, IRS Commissioner Everson said, "We see the twin cancers of technical manipulation and outright abuse that became evident in the profit-making sectors in the 1990s now migrating to too many pockets of the tax-exempt community."[12]

For their part, public charities and private foundations have sometimes offered inviting targets. The press has taken several high-profile offenders to task. The *Washington Post* ran an in-depth series on financial irregularities and conflicts of interest concerning loans and land deals at the Nature Conservancy, a $3-billion-plus environmental charity. Experts who deciphered the organization's tax returns and financial records called them "confounding" and akin to penetrating a "brick wall."[13] Elsewhere, the *Boston Globe* exposed the Paul & Virginia Cabot Charitable Trust, which reported 2002 assets of $5 million and made an average of $400,000 in yearly grants from 1998 to 2002 but paid trustee Paul Cabot Jr. more than $1.4 million. Cabot also used the trust's funds to cover mortgage payments on two homes, plus yacht and golf club bills.[14] Cabot was forced to repay more than $4 million to the family foundation under a deal struck with Massachusetts attorney general Thomas Reilly.

Public suspicion has been fueled by the attitude of many foundations. Until recently, many managed their affairs in ways that reinforced public perceptions of them as elite and opaque. They communicated little, if any, more than was legally required, failed to explain their mission or funding priorities, and neglected to seek objective appraisals of their grantmaking results. The field is moving away from this insular stance but foundations have considerable work to do to inform outside stakeholders of their missions and persuade them of their effectiveness and integrity.

This remoteness and mysteriousness may partly explain the erosion of public trust. In March 2004, the Philanthropic Initiative, a consulting group, held a forum on "Trust and Transparency: Philanthropy as Private Action in Public Space." Though participants felt that poor governance and accountability performance accounted in part for the loss of trust in philanthropy, they rated foundations' lack of transparency as the key contributing factor.[15]

Transparency has suffered on both sides of the information exchange equation. Most grantmakers perform poorly when it comes to sharing information about their objectives and their results. In 2003, for example, only 7 percent of the largest 20,000 foundations issued annual reports.[16] Moreover, until recently, there was little media attention to or public demand for news about philanthropy. What coverage there is tends to highlight alleged scandal or malfeasance, reinforcing the public's distrust of foundations. Although the spike in reported abuses might seem alarming, it still represents a minute proportion relative to the universe of foundations. Dorothy Ridings, who was then president and chief executive officer of the Council of Foundations, calls these offenders "a very tiny slice of foundation activity . . . a very visible, awful slice."[17]

Congress reacted to the spate of turn-of-the-twenty-first-century corporate governance and accounting scandals by passing the Sarbanes-Oxley Act of 2002. Sarbanes-Oxley mandates all publicly traded companies to include independent audit committees within their boards, have chief corporate officers certify financial statements, cut out insider loans, and strengthen whistle-blower protections. Although Congress has not formalized Sarbanes-Oxley–like mandates for charities, it seems to be getting close, or at least is encouraging the nonprofit sector to adopt some of the principles of transparency.

—w— Why the Attention Now?

During the summer of 2003, Congress reviewed foundation payout levels and administrative budgets as it debated the Charitable Giving Act, H.R. 7. The booming stock market of the 1990s grew the asset bases of American foundations considerably, spurring rises in overall grantmaking and increasing the prominence of foundations and their donors. Critics argued that foundations weren't giving away enough—that the annual minimum payout standard of 5 percent of assets was too low or that administrative expenses of grantmaking should be excluded from the payout equation. Watchdogs such as the National Committee for Responsive Philanthropy and the National Network of Grantmakers said foundations placed too high a premium on increasing and preserving their assets instead of spending more grant dollars to meet society's urgent needs *today,* sparking a vigorous debate about perpetuity and the present and future value of social investments.[18] Yet again, philanthropy was in a hot seat not experienced since the days of Wright Patman and the Tax Reform Act of 1969.

Although government has always overseen the nonprofit sector of which foundations are a part, there may be some reasons that regulators and legislators now appear to be focusing more intensively on this area. It is partly explained by the fact that the sector is growing ever larger, more complex, and more diverse, and the range of organizational forms, transactions, and practices that regulators must consider expands accordingly. In 1987, there were 1.3 million organizations in the entire nonprofit sector; a decade later, it encompassed 1.6 million, representing a 5 percent annual rate of increase.[19] Roughly half are tax-exempt 501(c)(3) public charities that file with the IRS.[20]

The ranks of foundations have ballooned in tandem with the overall growth of the nonprofit sector. From 1975 to 2002, the number of grant-making foundations roughly tripled, from 22,000 to 65,000. A statistic that may better signal their influence—and why regulators are apt to look more closely these days—is that their collective assets soared from $30 billion in 1975 to $435 billion now.[21]

In many areas, the lines among nonprofit, government, and business are blurring, particularly in fields such as health care and education, where charities frequently provide services also provided by government and commercial organizations. Hybrid organizations are more prevalent: some charities have formed for-profit ventures in one area that can be used to underwrite charitable services; other public charities provide services that look much like and compete with those provided by for-profit entities. These factors contribute, to varying degrees, to the shifting regulatory landscape that America's charities must navigate.

Regulating philanthropies has grown more complicated as well. Foundations used to be relatively uniform in type and operations, but now there are more diverse organizational forms within the field. Along with traditional grantmaking models, today there are venture philanthropies that partner so closely with nonprofits that it can get tough to tell where the funder's work ends and the grantee's begins. In health care, where many nonprofit hospitals and health plans had converted to for-profit status, a new breed of health philanthropy arose—the health care conversion foundation. Established with the proceeds from conversions, these foundations grew from 81 in 1997, with combined assets of $9.3 billion, to more than 170 in 2005 with $18.3 billion in assets.[22]

Donor-advised funds have also emerged as bold new players in philanthropy. Such funds have long been part of community foundations, but in the 1990s, many donor-advised funds were set up by commercial investment entities. Fidelity Investments led the way with its Charitable Gift Fund, and other banks and mutual funds companies have followed suit, attracting billions of investors' dollars that also flow to charitable causes. These new commercial donor-advised funds often compete with donor-advised funds operated by nonprofit community foundations and can be used by donors to avoid some of the inconvenience and restrictions of a private foundation. Policymakers are looking closely at whether or how to further regulate donor-advised funds.

Although this boom, even with the 2000–2003 downturn in assets, suggests that foundations are thriving as never before, it is precisely this rise in numbers, influence, and complexity, coupled with reductions in government spending for social services, that leaves them vulnerable to claims that they are "unaccountable."

At present, it is unclear how this current spate of legislative and regulatory review of charitable practices will shake out. Although some new requirements may be adopted, policymakers may decide that others are inappropriate or unnecessary. What is certain, however, is that leaders at foundations and charities of all sizes, from coast to coast, are feeling the heat of the spotlight from government and the media, and boardrooms are abuzz with talk about strengthening accountability and performance standards.

—〰— Philanthropy Responds

This current threat of regulation and legislation has prompted wide-ranging reactions among foundation and other nonprofit leaders. Some view any increase in government oversight as harmful and too intrusive, and believe the sector can regulate itself when it comes to public accountability.[23] Others claim it's high time for the government to put some enforcement muscle behind public expectations and that imposing Sarbanes-Oxley–like requirements would be the best way to ensure that charities can demostrate that they are honest, accountable stewards of the public's trust. Most leaders, not surprisingly, hold views that fall somewhere in the middle. They recognize that nonprofits must do more to show that they merit tax exemption and public support because they fulfill critical missions, perform valuable services, and adhere to high standards of performance and accountability. They believe that more effective regulation can support this goal.

The Council on Foundations, Independent Sector, the National Council of Nonprofit Associations, the National Committee for Responsive Philanthropy, and a host of other coordinating organizations have issued a call for all tax-exempt groups to demonstrate greater transparency, stronger accountability, and more rigorous governance. Though they have always encouraged nonprofits to pursue strong, ethical governance, they now frame these attributes as essential for the survival of charitable organizations in a hostile regulatory environment. The challenge for many of these organizations, such as the Council on Foundations and Independent Sector, is that their membership represents but a fraction of the 60,000-plus foundations and one-million-plus nonprofit organizations in the United States, and that they have little power, other than the power of persuasion, over their members' adherence to higher standards of accountability.

In 2004, the Council on Foundations launched "Building Strong and Ethical Foundations: Doing It Right," a nationwide governance and stewardship campaign. It calls upon foundations not only to comply with government regulations but also to uphold standards that may exceed legal requirements. It also is releasing a new publication called *Principles of Ethical Practice* for members and the field. Other national groups working to improve accountability and performance standards include the Better Business Bureau Wise Giving Alliance, GuideStar, and the Standards for Excellence Institute. GuideStar in particular has led the push for online reporting of charitable records, which vastly improves the accessibility of financial reports for donors and others. In partnership with the National Center for Charitable Statistics, GuideStar operates a free database that allows users to access IRS tax returns for more than a million charities, including foundations.[24]

Evidence suggests that this sectorwide push for demonstrated accountability may be taking hold. The Center for Effective Philanthropy, which surveyed the 250 largest philanthropies in 2004, found that foundation boards across the country were revisiting and fortifying governance practices. Two-thirds have discussed governance in the wake of recent corporate scandals and media attention to foundation operations, and 34 percent have approved changes.[25] Many of these changes involve foundations posting information on their Web sites—their tax returns, conflict of interest policies, codes of ethics, administrative expense ratios, even executive compensation schedules. This is meaningful progress.

Regional nonprofit and donor associations also are propelling improvements in governance and transparency. The Forum of Regional Associations of Grantmakers joined with PriceWaterhouseCoopers and the Charles Stewart Mott Foundation to publish no-nonsense guides to help funders submit more accurate and consistent tax returns to the IRS. They hope not just to drive up compliance rates but also to motivate grantmakers to use these forms as information tools that provide clear, usable data to the public and the press.[26]

Improving the quality of data reporting is no small feat. The Internal Revenue Service claims that paper filings of IRS Forms 990 and 990-PF show error rates of roughly 35 percent, including faulty, missing, or inconsistent data.[27] The Form 990-PF, which private foundations are required to file, lacks uniform standards and common definitions for reporting expenses. For instance, it does not allow funders to segregate those "administrative" expenses—such as staff-provided assistance to grantees, evaluations of grant programs, Web sites, and the production of an annual report—that promote effective and transparent philanthropy. Independent Sector's president, Diana Aviv, testified at the Finance Committee hearings that the existing forms "fall woefully short of providing a clear, useful tool for the public, for regulators, and for nonprofit practitioners."[28]

Regulators, meanwhile, are too poorly coordinated and underresourced to monitor charities' compliance effectively. Reviewing 990s for inaccuracies and other red flags has largely been beyond the reach of national and state regulators. The IRS Exempt Organizations division has lacked adequate staff and funding to police nonprofits. At the state level, oversight is even spottier. To further complicate matters, the tax code precludes state and IRS regulators from sharing information and collaborating on charity investigations. Although there was some momentum within the field to improve 990s prior to the Senate hearings, Independent Sector, foundation groups, and IRS officials are pressing ahead now with greater urgency to make them clearer, more transparent, and easier to file.

In September 2004, the Senate Finance Committee summoned Independent Sector to convene an independent national panel to recommend to Congress steps to "strengthen good governance, ethical conduct, and effective practice of public charities and private foundations." Paul Brest, president of the William and Flora Hewlett Foundation, and Cass Wheeler, CEO of the American Heart Association, lead this group of twenty-four charity and foundation executives, which looks like a fast-track version of the Filer Commission, which played such an important role in revamping the sector's practices in the 1970s. In June 2005, the Panel on the Nonprofit Sector issued its final recommendations to Congress to fortify accountability, transparency, and governance outcomes across America's nonprofit sector. While watchdog groups such as NCRP faulted the panel for recommending little more than stepped-up self-regulation, several key panel recommendations may hold promise for shoring up oversight of and confidence in nonprofits and foundations. Most notably, the report calls on Congress to allocate more resources to effective tax enforcement for and tracking of nonprofit groups and to appropriate federal dollars that help states do the same. It urges charities to disclose executive and trustee compensation levels and to keep those levels "reasonable," form clear conflict-of-interest and travel expense policies, be independently audited if annual revenues top $1 million or have a financial review performed by an independent accountant if they take in more than $250,000 but under $1 million, and require that at least one-third of all governing board members be independent. To improve foundation reporting, the panel calls for 990-PFs to draw bright, clear lines between grantmaking expenditures, program-related activities, administrative costs, and investments.[29]

The Senate Finance Committee is taking the more than one hundred suggestions of the panel under consideration as it weighs whether enhanced self-regulation by nonprofits and foundations will be sufficient to restore public confidence or if more legislative or regulatory guidance is needed.

—ɯ— The Robert Wood Johnson Foundation: How One Foundation Tackles the Accountability Challenge

In 1972, at the time the Robert Wood Johnson Foundation emerged as the nation's second-largest foundation, its sheer wealth made compliance with the 1969 Tax Reform Act a top priority. Foundation staff members immediately scrambled to develop policies and programs to get its first year's mandated payout—approximately $45 million—out the door. Executives soon sold off some Johnson & Johnson stock to meet the 20 percent ownership ceiling. At that time, they also worried about real or perceived governance conflicts; after all, Johnson & Johnson executives occupied half of the board seats. Gustav Lienhard, then the Foundation's president, delineated clear boundaries between Foundation and Johnson & Johnson operations, making it clear to the Foundation's staff, Johnson & Johnson, and external audiences that it was not the philanthropic wing of the corporation. The Foundation's leadership recognized that transparency and public accountability needed to be core operating principles in order to gain the trust of health leaders and public policymakers required to carry out its mission.

Though that initial urgency has dissipated over the years, Foundation leaders have continued to inculcate the founding board's belief that accountable management and effective governance demand persistent, deliberate effort. Trustees and executives regularly probe whether the Foundation is sufficiently rigorous in meeting performance and accountability benchmarks, and insist on a process of ongoing improvement. Such efforts help the institution to understand how well it is fulfilling its mission and demonstrating accountability to various stakeholders.

Board Governance

From the Robert Wood Johnson Foundation's earliest days, the board has met its fiduciary obligation, overseeing the Foundation's funds, policies, and practices entrusted to it for the benefit of the public. The Foundation's leadership is attentive to board composition; although it made sense in 1972 for Johnson & Johnson executives, who could channel Robert Wood Johnson's charitable interests, to occupy half of all board seats, today the proportion of those with ties to the company is about one-quarter. More important, trustees bring the financial management expertise, health and health care leadership, and policy perspectives needed to shape the Foundation's direction.[30]

One of the board's long-standing priorities has been to monitor the Foundation's performance in meeting its grantmaking objectives and responding to immediate and long-term issues in health and health care. Since 1992, one of the four annual board meetings has focused on assessing the Foundation's performance and accountability.

The Foundation's leaders have adopted data-driven tools to capture how well it serves the needs of various stakeholders. According to the Center for Effective Philanthropy, which published a case study on performance assessment at the Robert Wood Johnson Foundation, trustees and staff invest in assessment mechanisms that return a balanced, if imperfect, picture of the Foundation's performance and how well it addresses essential questions such as, What are we trying to accomplish? What are the results? How can we adjust goals to enhance impact?[31]

Administrative Cost Structure

For the past decade, the Foundation's administrative expenses, including compensation of staff, have typically fluctuated between 9 and 12 percent of its total costs of grantmaking. Because of the limitations of the IRS Form 990-PF that private foundations must file, most nongrant payments must be reported under the broad category of "operating and administrative expenses." Thus, the costs of certain major programs that are funded under contracts—such as the Covering Kids & Families campaign, a nationwide effort to promote the enrollment of eligible low-income children in governmental health insurance programs; the Center for Studying Health System Change, which tracks trends in the delivery and cost of health services and informs decision makers about them; and a broad-based national education campaign to improve end-of-life care in America—are considered by the IRS as operating and administrative expenses.

Even though they are reported as "operating and administrative expenses," contractual arrangements such as these are viewed by Foundation board members and staff as efficient means of improving health and health care.

That said, the Foundation is working to cut back on administrative expenses by closely managing travel costs, trimming the use of consultants, and streamlining processes across departments. Given its breadth of operations and its commitment to providing technical assistance to grantees, however, it is unlikely that the Foundation will find itself on the lower end of the administrative cost scale anytime soon.

Evaluation and Communications: Assessing and Reporting Successes, Failures, and Lessons Learned

The Robert Wood Johnson Foundation has been evaluating grants and programs for almost as long as it has funded them. National initiatives, as a general rule, are evaluated by outside experts, ranging from leading academicians to staff members of research firms to experienced health care practitioners. Evaluators are given wide latitude to select state-of-the-art methods and to come to independent conclusions about impact. Two rationales motivate the Foundation's work in this area: evaluation informs key decisions to improve health and health care for Americans, and it helps the Foundation shape future programs.

In addition to formal program evaluations, the Foundation assesses impact through three other approaches: (1) the annual *Robert Wood Johnson Foundation Anthology*, which synthesizes findings from the Foundation's grantmaking areas, (2) Grants Results Reports, which summarize findings from specific grants and national programs, and (3) a performance appraisal system, which tracks the Foundation's progress in meeting its short-, medium-, and long-term objectives.

The Foundation also seeks to get a fuller, clearer picture of the impact and the quality of its work by asking internal and external audiences a fundamental question: How are we doing? Answers to that core question come through a variety of channels, primarily from its annual "scorecard." In addition to containing case studies and performance measures designed to show progress, or lack thereof, toward reaching the objectives established by the Foundation, the scorecard also asks key constituents for their assessment of whether the Foundation is focusing its programs on the right issues and whether it is effective. It asks grantees, potential grantees, and applicants whose proposals were turned down how fair and responsive the staff is to applicants and grantees and whether policymakers, opinion leaders, and journalists know about the Foundation and find its work useful. It also asks staff members what they think of the Foundation as a place to work. Each July, the Foundation's trustees use the scorecard to assess organizational performance and to set goals for the institution.

In 2004, the Foundation complemented its own survey by asking the Center for Effective Philanthropy to conduct an in-depth analysis of its performance and responsiveness through the eyes of its grantees. The Center for Effective Philanthropy compared responses from 200 of the Foundation's grantees with those of more than 3,500 grantees of twenty-nine other foundations. The Foundation rated relatively poorly in customer satisfaction, fairness and responsiveness, clarity of funding priorities, and grantee selection criteria. In a commentary e-mailed to national program directors, the Foundation's president and CEO, Risa Lavizzo-Mourey, called the findings "sobering, to put it mildly."

The results from the Center for Effective Philanthropy survey have driven an intense examination of the Foundation's internal grantmaking and administrative processes. In 2004, the Foundation initiated a top-to-bottom review of its grantmaking practices to remedy many of the problems that had been identified, align them more closely with the expectations of the field, and be clearer in communicating about program objectives. These are essential steps in the Foundation's continuing quest to be a more effective and accountable philanthropy.

The Foundation not only evaluates its programs, its grantmaking, and its staff's performance; it also places high priority on communicating with the field, policymakers, and the public. It publicizes not just the glowing successes but also the disappointments and everything in between, sharing lessons from each outcome. Outcomes and results are shared through the *Anthology, Advances* (the Foundation's quarterly newsletter), the *Annual Report,* special reports, a new Web-based research center, and Grants Results Reports. At present, there are approximately 1,400 reports on projects and more than sixty reports on national programs posted on the Grants Results Reporting section of the Foundation's Web site.

The Foundation has learned that evaluation and communications work hand in hand in fostering greater transparency and driving social change. Over time, the Foundation has placed a high priority on strategic communications. Communications are an integral part of the Foundation's grantmaking approaches, and communications strategies sometimes form the crux of grant programs that foster Foundation goals, such as promoting access to health care (the Covering Kids campaign) or reducing harm caused by substance use (the Campaign for Tobacco-Free Kids). In 2004, communications grants made up roughly 19 percent of the funds awarded by the Foundation. The Foundation also helps grantees build their outreach capacity so that they may communicate the results of their work effectively to key audiences.[32]

In addition to advancing the Foundation's grantmaking practice and performance, the way in which it combines evaluation and communications also provides tangible evidence of the Foundation's commitment to be accountable and transparent. It informs the efforts of those working in health, health care, and social change, and in a wider sense provides a base of evidence for policymakers, the media, and the public increasingly seeking proof that public charities and foundations add value to society.

—⁓— Closing the Performance and Perception Gap

Private foundations are unique: they command tremendous financial resources intended for the public good, yet they typically are unconstrained by the accountability systems that drive government, the financial bottom line of commercial enterprises, and the need for funds or the competition for service recipients that increasingly motivates other types of charitable organizations. Peter Karoff, a consultant, calls American philanthropy "the largest pool of private capital available in the world that is free from the constraints of governments or the marketplace."[33]

Foundations and other charitable organizations seem to be at a crossroads. All signs suggest that the accountability bar has been raised; it is now their responsibility to figure out how to clear it. In 2003 and 2004, Congress teetered at the edge of passing new laws to force charities to adhere to more stringent governance and accountability standards. California and Massachusetts already have enacted tougher reporting requirements, and other states and the federal government may follow their lead. The potential is there for such measures to constrain the way nonprofits do their work; for small charities in particular, they can pose backbreaking compliance burdens. Clearly, if foundations and other charities fail to strengthen their governance practices and their accountability, they face the unpalatable prospect of government imposing them from outside.

Regardless of how policymakers ultimately address this dilemma, the move toward stronger standards of ethics, accountability, transparency, and governance will have beneficial long-term outcomes for foundations. Philanthropy is likely to grow at a fast pace; researchers predict that the economy will be infused with $41 trillion in new wealth over the next fifty years, coming primarily from the estates of aging baby boomers.[34] This influx holds great promise for expanding Americans' philanthropic giving and enhancing the impact of the foundation sector. If this growth is marked by sustained emphasis on accountability, foundations should emerge as stronger organizations that enjoy public support for their role as stewards of private wealth for public good.

Glossary

Form 990: The annual tax return that tax-exempt organizations with gross revenue of more than $25,000 must file with the IRS. The Form 990 also is generally filed with the appropriate state offices. This return includes information about the organization's assets, income, operating expenses, contributions, paid staff and salaries, names and addresses of persons to contact, and program areas.

Form 990-PF: The annual information return that must be filed with the IRS by private foundations and nonexempt charitable trusts that are treated as private foundations by the IRS.

Foundation: A nongovernmental charitable nonprofit corporation or trust with funds and a program managed by its trustees or directors, established to further social, educational, religious, or charitable activities, often by making grants. A private foundation receives its funds from, and often is controlled by, an individual, family, corporation, or other group consisting of a limited number of members. In contrast, a community foundation receives its funds from multiple donors and is classified by the IRS as a public charity.

Independent sector: The portion of the economy that includes all 501(c)(3) charitable and 501(c)(4) social welfare tax-exempt organizations as defined by the IRS, including all religious institutions (such as churches and synagogues). The independent sector is also referred to as the "voluntary sector," the "nonprofit sector," and the "third sector."

Nonprofit: A term describing a charitable trust or a nonprofit corporation that has no shareholders or other owners and that does not distribute dividends or other earnings. A nonprofit organization's income is used to support its operations. Nonprofit organizations that are included in the definition of the independent sector are nonprofit, tax-exempt organizations that are included in sections 501(c)(3) and 501(c)(4) of the code.

Payout requirement: The Internal Revenue Code requirement that all private foundations, including corporate foundations, pay out annually in grants and related expenditures the equivalent of 5 percent of the value of their investment assets.

Public charity: The largest category of 501(c)(3) organizations, which serve broad purposes, including assisting the poor and the underprivileged; advancing religion, education, health, science, art, and culture; and protecting the environment, among other purposes. A charity qualifies as a public charity by virtue of its activities or broad public support. Churches, educational institutions, and hospitals are considered public charities based on their activities. Other public charities, such as United Way–type organizations or museums, qualify by receiving a substantial part of their income, directly or indirectly, from the general public or from government sources. The public support must be fairly broad and not limited to a few individuals or families. Charities that do not meet the activity or public support tests are known as private foundations under Section 509(a) of the Internal Revenue Code.

Section 501(c)(3): The Internal Revenue Code section that defines tax-exempt organizations organized and operated exclusively for religious, charitable, scientific, literary, educational, or similar purposes. Contributions to 501(c)(3) organizations are deductible as charitable donations for federal income tax purposes. These organizations make up a large part of the independent sector.

Section 501(c)(4): The Internal Revenue Code section that defines tax-exempt organizations organized to operate as civic leagues, social welfare organizations, and local associations of employees. Contributions to 501(c)(4) organizations are not deductible as charitable donations for federal income tax purposes. Section 501(c)(4) organizations are considered part of the independent sector.

Tax-exempt: A classification under Section 501(c) of the Internal Revenue Code for qualified nonprofit organizations that excludes their income from federal income tax. There are twenty-eight categories of tax-exempt entities; 501(c)(3) and 501(c)(4) organizations are two of them. Although private foundations, including company foundations, are tax-exempt, they must pay a 1 or 2 percent excise tax on net investment income.

Excerpted from Independent Sector and the Urban Institute. *The New Nonprofit Almanac and Desk Reference.* San Francisco: Jossey-Bass, 2002. Brought up to date by the general counsel's office of the Robert Wood Johnson Foundation.

Notes

1. Federal News Service Transcript. "Charity Oversight and Reform: Keeping Bad Things from Happening to Good Charities." Remarks by Sen. Chuck Grassley at U.S. Senate Committee on Finance Hearing, June 22, 2004.

2. Internal Revenue Service. "IRS Initiative Will Scrutinize EO Compensation Practices." News release issued August 10, 2004. (http://www.irs.gov/newsroom/article/0,,id=128328,00.html).

3. California Registry of Charitable Trusts. "Nonprofit Integrity Act of 2004: Summary of Key Provisions." 2004. (http://caag.state.ca.us/charities/publications/nonprofit_integrity_act_summary_oct04.pdf).

4. National Council of Nonprofit Associations. "Nonprofit Oversight and Accountability Proposals and Bills Introduced at the State Level, 2005." (http://www.ncna.org/_uploads/documents/live//2005_State_Governance-Updated_6-20-2005.doc); Minnesota House of Representatives. "H.F. No. 593, as introduced—84th Legislative Session." 2005. (http://www.revisor.leg.state.mn.us/bin/bldbill.php?bill=H0593.0&session=ls84); and "H.F. No. 961, as introduced—84th Legislative Session." (http://www.revisor.leg.state.mn.us/bin/bldbill.php?bill=H0961.0&session=ls84).

5. Davis, M., Jr., and Weiss, B. "When Bad Things Happened to a Good Foundation." *Foundation News & Commentary,* Sept.–Oct. 2004, pp. 17–20.

6. Greene, S. G. "Former Irvine Foundation CEO and His Wife Repay Fund for Benefits That Raised Questions." *The Chronicle of Philanthropy,* January 8, 2004. (http://philanthropy.com/premium/articles/v16/i06/06004302.htm).

7. Wirthlin Worldwide. "2003 Congressional and Public Opinions of Private Foundations." Report prepared for the Council on Foundations, "National Quorum Interview Schedule," 2003.

8. Kiger, J. C. *Philanthropic Foundations in the Twentieth Century.* Westport, Conn.: Greenwood Press, 2000, pp. 23–24.

9. Labovitz, J. R. "1969 Tax Reforms Reconsidered." *The Future of Foundations.* Englewood Cliffs, N.J.: Prentice-Hall, 1973, pp. 101–102; Troyer, T. A. "The Cataclysm of '69." *Foundation News & Commentary,* March-April 1999, pp. 40–47.

10. Internal Revenue Service. "Testimony: Charitable Giving Problems." 2004. (http://www.irs.gov/newsroom/article/0,,id=124203,00.html).

11. Light, P. C. "Fact Sheet on the Continued Crisis in Charitable Confidence." 2004. (http://www.brook.edu/dybdocroot/views/papers/light/20040913.pdf); "Trust in Charitable Organizations." Brooking Institution Policy Brief. 2002. (http://www.brook.edu/comm/reformwatch/rw06.pdf).

12. Everson, M. Plenary Speech at the Annual Conference of the Council on Foundations, April 12, 2005. (http://www.cof.org/files/Documents/Government/05_AC_Mark_Everson_Speech_Transcription.doc).

13. Stephens, J., and Ottaway, D. B. "IRS to Audit Nature Conservancy from Inside." *Washington Post,* January 17, 2004, A01.

14. Robinson, W., and Rezendes, M. "Foundation Chief Agrees to Pay Over $4M." *Boston Globe.* December 16, 2004, p. A1; Healy, B., Latour, F., Pfeiffer, S., Rezendes, M., and Robinson, W. "Some Officers of Charities Steer Assets to Selves." *Boston Globe.* October 9, 2003, p. A1.

15. The Philanthropic Initiative. "On the Issue of Trust." *INITIATIVES: A Newsletter on Strategic Philanthropy.* May 2004. (http://www.tpi.org/promoting/publications/init/May2004_trust.pdf).

16. Georgetown University. "Governance and Accountability in America's Foundations." Transcript from the Center for Public and Nonprofit Leadership Issues Forum. January 29, 2004. (http://cpnl.georgetown.edu/doc_pool/lF01Governance.pdf).

17. Ridings, D. S. "Foundations' Hidden Treasures." *Foundation News & Commentary,* Sept.–Oct., 2004, p. 15.

18. Klausner, M. "When Time Isn't Money: Foundation Payouts and the Time Value of Money." *Stanford Social Innovation Review.* Spring 2003, pp. 50–59; Strom, S. "Foundations Roiled by Measure to Spur Increase in Charity." *New York Times.* May 19, 2003, p. A1.

19. Independent Sector and the Urban Institute. *The New Nonprofit Almanac & Desk Reference.* San Francisco: Jossey-Bass, 2002. (http://www.urban.org/UploadedPDF/AlmanacExSum.pdf).

20. Urban Institute. National Center for Charitable Statistics. "Number of Nonprofit Organizations in the United States 1996–2004." (http://nccsdataweb.urban.org/PubApps/profile1.php?state=US).

21. Foundation Center. "Number of Grantmaking Foundations, Assets, Total Giving and Gifts Received, 1975 to 2002." 2002. (http://fdncenter.org/fc_stats/pdf/02_found_growth/04_02.pdf).

22. Grantmakers in Health. "The Business of Giving." 2005. Washington, D.C.: GIH, 2005.

23. Meyerson, A. "A Serious Threat to Philanthropic Freedom." *Philanthropy,* July-Aug. 2004, pp. 2–3.

24. Even though foundations are considered tax-exempt organizations, they must file a tax return, Form 990-PF, with the IRS and usually also with the states in which they are incorporated.

25. The Center for Effective Philanthropy. "Foundation Governance: The CEO Viewpoint." 2004. (http://www.effectivephilanthropy.com/images/pdfs/governanceceoview.pdf).

26. Gallagher, M. "Foundations Strive for Accountability And Transparency Through 990-PFs." Press release issued by the Council of Michigan Foundations, June 2, 2004. (http:www.cmif.org/News_Detailed.asp?ID=496).

27. Williams, G. "Government Requires Electronic Filing." *The Chronicle of Philanthropy,* January 20, 2005. (http://philanthropy.com/premium/articles/v17/i07/07003902.htm).

28. Independent Sector. "Testimony of Diana Aviv, President and CEO, Independent Sector." Provided for U.S. Senate Committee on Finance Hearing, June 22, 2004. (http://finance.senate.gov/hearings/testimony/2004test/062204datest.pdf).

29. Panel on the Nonprofit Sector. "Strengthening Transparency, Governance, Accountability of Charitable Organizations: A Final Report to Congress and

the Nonprofit Sector." June 2005. (http://www.nonprofitpanel.org/final/Panel_Final_Report.pdf).

30. For the depth of field-specific skill and knowledge they deliver, plus the substantial time they give in carrying out their duties, the Robert Wood Johnson Foundation compensates its trustees modestly for their service.

31. Giudice, P., and Bolduc, K. *Assessing Performance at the Robert Wood Johnson Foundation: A Case Study.* Boston, Mass.: The Center for Effective Philanthropy, 2004.

32. Karel, F. "Getting the Word Out: A Foundation Memoir and Personal Journey." *To Improve Health and Health Care 2001: The Robert Wood Johnson Foundation Anthology.* San Francisco: Jossey-Bass, 2001.

33. Karoff, H. P. "Introduction: Serious Travelers." *Just Money: A Critique of Contemporary American Philanthropy.* Boston: TPI Editions, 2004, p. xv.

34. Center on Wealth and Philanthropy. "The Markets May Be Down, But the Largest Intergenerational Transfer of Wealth in History Is Still Coming to Town." Boston College, 2003. (http://www.bc.edu/research/swri/meta-elements/pdf/41trillionpressrelease.pdf).

-ᴍ-The Editors

Stephen L. Isaacs, J.D., is a partner in Isaacs/Jellinek, a San Francisco–based consulting firm, and president of Health Policy Associates, Inc. A former professor of public health at Columbia University and founding director of its Development Law and Policy Program, he has written extensively for professional and popular audiences. His book *The Consumer's Legal Guide to Today's Health Care* was reviewed as "the single best guide to the health care system in print today." His articles have been widely syndicated and have appeared in law reviews and health policy journals. He also provides technical assistance internationally on health law, civil society, and social policy. A graduate of Brown University and Columbia Law School, Isaacs served as vice president of International Planned Parenthood's Western Hemisphere Region, practiced health law, and spent four years in Thailand as a program officer for the U.S. Agency for International Development.

James R. Knickman, Ph.D., is vice president for research and evaluation at the Robert Wood Johnson Foundation. He oversees a range of grants and national programs supporting research and policy analysis to better understand forces that can improve health status and delivery of health care. In addition, he is in charge of developing formal evaluations of national programs supported by the Foundation. During the 1999–2000 academic year, he held a Regents' Lectureship at the University of California, Berkeley. Previously, Knickman was on the faculty of the Robert Wagner Graduate School of Public Service at New York University. At NYU, he was the founding director of a university-wide research center focused on urban health care. His publications include research on a range of health care topics, with particular emphasis on issues related to financing and delivering long-term care. He has served on numerous health-related advisory committees at the state and local levels and spent a year working at New York City's Office of Management and Budget. Currently, he chairs the board of trustees of Robert Wood Johnson University Hospital in New Brunswick. He completed his undergraduate work at Fordham University and received his doctorate in public policy analysis from the University of Pennsylvania.

–ᴡ–The Contributors

James Bornemeier is a writer with twenty-five years experience in journalism as an editor and correspondent at the *Los Angeles Times, Philadelphia Inquirer,* and *Providence Journal.* He is now editorial director of a law firm in New York City. Previously, he was a writing and editing consultant, working primarily with major charitable organizations such as the Ford Foundation, the Robert Wood Johnson Foundation, and the Goldman Sachs Foundation. From 1997 to 2003, he worked as public affairs officer at The Pew Charitable Trusts, where he oversaw communications for the culture and public policy programs. He is a graduate of Northwestern University.

Paul Brodeur was a staff writer at *The New Yorker* for many years. During that time, he alerted the nation to the public health hazard posed by asbestos, to depletion of the ozone layer by chlorofluorocarbons, and to the harmful effects of microwave radiation and power-frequency electromagnetic fields. His work has been acknowledged with a National Magazine Award and the Journalism Award of the American Association for the Advancement of Science. The United Nations Environment Program has named him to its Global 500 Roll of Honour for outstanding environmental achievements.

Victor A. Capoccia is a senior program officer at the Robert Wood Johnson Foundation, where he leads the addiction prevention and treatment team, and also focuses on developing skills and career paths for frontline health and health care workers. A former chief executive officer and president of CAB Health and Recovery Services, Inc., a community-based treatment and prevention agency, and director of community health services, the city health agency of the Boston Department of Health and Hospitals, he also served on the Institute of Medicine Committee on Community-Based Drug Treatment, and chaired the Center for Substance Abuse Treatment Panel on Improving and Strengthening Treatment Systems. As associate professor in community organization and social planning at Boston College Graduate School of Social Work, he conducted research and published articles on the changing responsibility and roles of local, state, and federal government to provide health and social services to vulnerable populations. A graduate of Boston College, he holds master's degrees in social work and city planning and a doctorate in social policy from the Florence Heller Graduate School of Social Welfare at Brandeis. Capoccia has served on boards of community health planning, housing, and civic organizations, as well as worked in Community Action and Model Cities programs.

Digby Diehl is a writer, literary collaborator, and television, print, and Internet journalist. Recently honored with the Jack Smith Award from the Friends of the Pasadena Public Library, his book credits include *Angel on My Shoulder,* the autobiography of singer Natalie Cole; *The Million Dollar Mermaid,* the autobiography of MGM star Esther Williams; *Tales from the Crypt,* the history of the popular comic book, movie, and television series; and *A Spy for All Seasons,* the autobiography of former CIA officer Duane Clarridge. For eleven years, Diehl was the literary correspondent for ABC-TV's "Good Morning America," and he was recently the book editor for the "Home Page" show on MSNBC. He continues to appear regularly on the morning news on KTLA. Previously the entertainment editor for KCBS television in Los Angeles, he was a writer for the Emmys and for the soap opera "Santa Barbara," book editor of the *Los Angeles Herald Examiner,* editor in chief of art book publisher Harry N. Abrams, and the founding book editor of the *Los Angeles Times Book Review.* Diehl holds an M.A. in theater from UCLA and a B.A. in American studies from Rutgers University, where he was a Henry Rutgers Scholar.

Marsha R. Gold is a senior fellow at Mathematica Policy Research, Inc., where she conducts research focused on managed care and the translation of research into practice. In the area of Medicaid managed care, she has conducted national surveys of plans to learn about the characteristics of provider networks, payment policy, and quality improvement activities, developing analytical frameworks to help policymakers evaluate and improve access to physician services, and case studies of leading state initiatives. She has published widely in peer-review journals, sits on the boards of *Health Affairs* and *Health Services Research,* and serves as an expert resource for policymakers, other researchers, and the media. Before joining Mathematica in 1992, she was director of research and analysis for the Group Health Association of America and director of policy analysis and program evaluation in the secretary's office at the Maryland Department of Health and Mental Hygiene. Mathematica, an employee-owned firm, with offices in Princeton, New Jersey, Washington, D.C., and Cambridge, Massachusetts, has conducted some of the most important evaluations of health care, education, welfare, employment, nutrition, and early childhood programs and policies in the United States.

Susan Krutt is a communications associate for the Robert Wood Johnson Foundation's health group, working with the childhood obesity, tobacco, and public health teams. She also helps manage cross-cutting initiatives at the Foundation, including the television health series and the sports philanthropy project. Prior to joining the Foundation in December 2002, she was a research associate with the Annenberg Public Policy Center at the University of Pennsylvania and a summer associate in the public policy program of the Pew Charitable Trusts. She also managed communications efforts for the Aspen Institute's Nonprofit Sector & Philanthropy Program in Washington, D.C., where she worked for five years. Krutt received her M.A. from the University of Pennsylvania's Annenberg School for Communication and her B.A. in international relations from Colgate University.

Risa Lavizzo-Mourey is the fourth president and chief executive officer of the Robert Wood Johnson Foundation, a position she assumed in January 2003. Under her leadership, the Foundation implemented a defining framework that focuses its mission to improve the health and health care of all Americans and set bold objectives in nursing, health care disparities, and childhood obesity, as well as improving public health and quality in the health care system. She originally joined the staff in April 2001 as the senior vice president and director, health care group. Prior to coming to the Foundation, Lavizzo-Mourey was the Sylvan Eisman Professor of Medicine and Health Care Systems at the University of Pennsylvania, as well as director of the Institute on Aging. Lavizzo-Mourey was the deputy administrator of the Agency for Health Care Policy and Research, now known as the Agency for Health Care Research and Quality. Lavizzo-Mourey is the author of numerous articles and several books, the recipient of many awards and honorary doctorates, and frequently appears on national radio and television. A member of the Institute of Medicine of the National Academy of Sciences, she earned her medical degree at Harvard Medical School, followed by a master's in business administration at the University of Pennsylvania's Wharton School. After completing a residency in internal medicine at Brigham and Women's Hospital in Boston, Massachusetts, Lavizzo-Mourey was a Robert Wood Johnson Clinical Scholar at the University of Pennsylvania, where she also received her geriatrics training.

Jane Isaacs Lowe is a senior program officer at the Robert Wood Johnson Foundation and serves as the team leader for the vulnerable populations portfolio, a program staff group focused on improving social-health outcomes for low-income children, families, and older adults. At the Foundation, she is also responsible for the development of minority health professions training programs and a matching grants program with local funding partners. She is currently a fellow at the New York Academy of Medicine, and the president of the board of Grantmakers in Aging. Lowe came to the Foundation from the University of Pennsylvania School of Social Work, where she served as member of the faculty (1989–1998). She was the recipient of the Outstanding Teaching Award in 1992 and 1997. From 1976 to 1989, she worked at the Mt. Sinai Medical Center (New York City), where she served as a faculty member in the medical school's department of community medicine and as a hospital social work administrator. Lowe has extensive experience in chronic illness, community-based health, and program planning. She earned her bachelor's degree in sociology and education from Cedar Crest College, her master's degree in social work from Columbia University, and her doctorate in social welfare policy and planning from Rutgers University.

Geralyn Graf Magan is a freelance writer based in Maryland. A former newspaper reporter, she has been writing about issues affecting older people for almost thirty years. For more than a decade, she wrote *Housing Report* for the AARP, and now writes various AARP publications and Web articles for and about grandparents raising grandchildren. She recently developed a comprehensive Web feature on universal design for AARP. In 2002, she authored *Communicating with the 50+ Audience About Physical Activity Issues* and coauthored *The Role of Midlife and Older Consumers in Promoting Physical Activity Through Health Care Settings.*

Robin E. Mockenhaupt is the deputy director for the health group at the Robert Wood Johnson Foundation. Areas of current investment in the health group include childhood obesity, public health, tobacco, and addiction prevention and treatment. Formerly, she served as a senior program officer, from 1999–2003, and she worked on health behavior, physical activity, and chronic disease management issues. Before joining the Foundation in September 1999, Mockenhaupt worked in the field services department at AARP in Washington, D.C. Prior to that, she held positions in other departments at AARP, including field operations manager of Health Advocacy Services, and was director of the National Resource Center on Health Promotion and Aging. She has also held positions at Focus Technologies, Inc., in Washington, D.C.; the National Center for Education in Maternal and Child Health, Georgetown University; and the National Health Screening Council, Bethesda, Maryland. She is coauthor of the book, *Healthy Aging,* along with Kathleen Boyle. Mockenhaupt received a Ph.D. in health education from the University of Maryland, a graduate certificate in gerontology from the Center on Aging at the University of Maryland, an M.P.H. in health administration and health education from Columbia University, and a B.S. in biology from Pennsylvania State University.

David Morse is vice president for communications at the Robert Wood Johnson Foundation. From 1997 to 2001, he was director of public affairs for the Pew Charitable Trusts, responsible for managing the Trusts' relationships with media and policymakers and with advising grantees on communications strategies. Before joining Pew, Morse served as associate vice president for policy planning at the University of Pennsylvania, building the university's relations with the federal government, leading efforts to create new mechanisms for financing higher education, and promoting tax policies that preserve incentives for charitable giving. As an aide to U.S. Senators Jacob Javits and Robert Stafford, Morse developed legislation affecting higher education and cultural affairs for the Senate Committee on Labor and Human Resources, and in 1981 directed the President's Task Force on the Arts and the Humanities. He received a B.A. from Hamilton College and an M.A. from the Johns Hopkins University. He serves on the board of the Communications Network and on the Ad Council's Public Policy Advisory Committee, and from 1994 to 2001 taught a public policy course at the University of Pennsylvania's Graduate School of Education.

Robert Rosenblatt is a senior fellow at the National Academy of Social Insurance (NASI), a nonpartisan think tank providing information on Social Security, Medicare, and related programs. This is one of his activities as a freelance writer and editor specializing in policy issues of the aging society, including retirement and health care. He also writes a column on health policy issues for the Web site of the California HealthCare Foundation. Previously, he was a Washington correspondent for the *Los Angeles Times,* where he covered economics, financial issues, and health care policy and helped create the paper's first beat specializing in aging stories. He also wrote a column on health insurance benefits for the *Los Angeles Times* health care section. He is a winner of the Loeb award for financial journalism. Rosenblatt has a B.A. in economics from City College of New York and an M.S. in journalism from the Columbia School of Journalism.

Erin Fries Taylor is a health researcher at Mathematica Policy Research. Her research interests include access to care and quality-related issues for uninsured and low-income persons. Taylor also has a strong interest in Medicare policy; her dissertation research analyzed the variation in

Medicare supplemental coverage across geographic markets. She has published in *Health Affairs, Health Services Research,* and *Journal of Health Economics.* Prior to graduate school, Taylor worked as a research economist at the Research Triangle Institute and Triangle Economic Research in the Raleigh-Durham area of North Carolina. Taylor has a Ph.D. from the University of Michigan and an undergraduate degree from the College of William and Mary.

Justin S. White is currently a graduate student at the University of North Carolina's School of Public Health and contributed to this volume while working as an analyst at Mathematica Policy Research. His research at Mathematica focused largely on Medicaid, including Medicaid managed care, mental health services utilization, and state Medicaid buy-in programs. He has published in *Health Affairs.* White holds a bachelor's degree from Bucknell University.

Irene M. Wielawski is a health care journalist with twenty years' experience as a staff writer for daily newspapers, including the *Providence Journal-Bulletin* and the *Los Angeles Times,* where she was a member of the investigations team. She has written extensively on problems of access to care among the poor and uninsured, and other socioeconomic issues in American medicine. From 1994 through 2000, Wielawski—with a research grant from the Robert Wood Johnson Foundation—tracked the experiences of the medically uninsured in twenty-five states following the demise of President Clinton's health reform plan. Other projects in health care journalism since then include helping to develop a pediatric medicine program for public television, as well as freelance writing and editing for various publications, including the *New York Times, Los Angeles Times,* and science and policy journals. Wielawski has been a finalist for the Pulitzer Prize for medical reporting, among other solo honors. She is a founder of the Association of Health Care Journalists and a graduate of Vassar College.

–ᴡ–Index

Institute for the Future of Aging Services, 55
Institute of Medicine (IOM), 37, 82, 83, 86, 89, 142, 152
Interfaith Volunteer Caregivers Program, 202–204
Internal Revenue Code, 218–219; definitions in, 238–239
Internal Revenue Service (IRS), 17, 223–224, 225, 230–231
Internal Revenue Service (IRS) tax returns: improving the quality of, 230–231; publicizing of, 229; Tax Reform Act on, 222
IRS Form 990, 230–231, 237
IRS Form 990-PF, 230–231, 237
Investment risk regulation, 222
Irvine Foundation, 218
Islamic Society of North America, 204
Issue portfolios, 92–93
Istook, E., 224

J

James Irvine Foundation, 218
Jellinek, P., 89–90, 106, 107*n*.10, 192, 205, 210*n*.2*n*.13
Joanou, P., 147
John R. Wooden High School, 170
Johns Hopkins Medical Institutions, 193, 194–195
Johnson, K., 203
Johnson, L. B., 71
Johnson, N. L., 20–21
Johnson & Johnson, 194, 232–233
Join Together, 149, 156
Join Together On Line, 149
Jones, J., 7, 10
Journal of the American Medical Society, 100
Just Say No campaign, 144

K

Kahekili Terrace, 21–23
Kahn, C., 76
Kahn, R. L., 36, 59*n*.5
Kaiser, H. J., 72
Kaiser clinics, 72
Kaiser Permanente, 122
Karel, F., 193, 199, 242*n*.32
Karoff, H. P., 236, 242*n*.33
Kaufman, N., 9, 207, 208

Keenan, P., 191
Keenan, T., 107*n*.10, 174; background, activities, and influence of, 187–210; at Commonwealth Fund, 192–194; as consultant to Robert Wood Johnson Foundation, 189; early life and education of, 191–192; and interfaith caregiving programs, 202–205; and Local Initiative Funding Partners Program, 198–202; networking of, 209; and nurses' training, 205–209; philanthropic approach of, 187–188, 190–191, 198–199, 206–207, 209–210; *The Promise at Hand* by, 190–191; retirement of, 189; at Robert Wood Johnson Foundation, 194–210
Keenan Leadership Award in Health Philanthropy, 209
Kennedy, E. M., 79, 89
Kennedy, J. F., 71
Kenneson, M., 137*n*.15
Kentucky Department of Education, 5
Kentucky Frontier Nursing Service, 207
Kevitt, M., 60*n*.20
Keystone Mercy Health Plan, 181
Kiger, J. C., 240*n*.8
King, S., 20, 21
King Foundation, 217–218
Kingston Hospital, New York, 203
Kinsella, K., 59*n*.7, *n*.16
Klausner, M., 241*n*.18
Kovar, P. A., 60*n*.19
Kovner, A. R., 107*n*.5
Krutt, S., 213, 214, 215

L

Labovitz, J. R., 240*n*.9
Laidlaw Transit Services, 173
Landon, B. E., 136*n*.12, *n*.4
Larios, P., 181
Lavizzo-Mourey, R., 92–93, 106–107, 154, 209–210, 235
LeRoy, L., 209
Lester, M., 14–15, 16
Liebe, R., 13
Lienhard, G., 194, 232
Life Options, 42
Light, P., 224–225, 240*n*.11
Lobbying, 221–222

–ɯ–Table of Contents
To Improve Health and Health Care 1997

–ᵐ–Table of Contents

To Improve Health and Health Care 1998–1999

–ɯ–Table of Contents

To Improve Health and Health Care 2000

—ⅲ—Table of Contents

To Improve Health and Health Care 2001

–ɯ–Table of Contents

To Improve Health and Health Care Volume V

–ɰ–Table of Contents

To Improve Health and Health Care Volume VI

~ɯ~Table of Contents
To Improve Health and Health Care Volume VII

~ɯ~Table of Contents

To Improve Health and Health Care Volume VIII